# Botanical Defenders: Herbal Antivirals Unveiled

### Harnessing Nature's Immune-Boosting Power

## Lauren Hayes

© **Copyright 2024 - All rights reserved.**

The content contained within this book may not be reproduced, duplicated or transmitted without direct written permission from the author or the publisher.

Under no circumstances will any blame or legal responsibility be held against the publisher, or author, for any damages, reparation, or monetary loss due to the information contained within this book, either directly or indirectly.

**Legal Notice:**

This book is copyright protected. It is only for personal use. You cannot amend, distribute, sell, use, quote or paraphrase any part, or the content within this book, without the consent of the author or publisher.

**Disclaimer Notice:**

Please note the information contained within this document is for educational and entertainment purposes only. All effort has been executed to present accurate, up to date, reliable, complete information. No warranties of any kind are declared or implied. Readers acknowledge that the author is not engaging in the rendering of legal, financial, medical or professional advice. The content within this book has been derived from various sources. Please consult a licensed professional before attempting any techniques outlined in this book.

By reading this document, the reader agrees that under no circumstances is the author responsible for any losses, direct or indirect, that are incurred as a result of the use of information contained within this document, including, but not limited to, errors, omissions, or inaccuracies.

# Table of Contents

**INTRODUCTION** .................................................................. 6
**CHAPTER I: The Foundations of Herbal Antivirals** ............ 8
  Historical Use of Herbs for Immune Support ..................... 8
  Science Behind Herbal Antiviral Properties ...................... 10
  Differentiating Herbal Antivirals from Traditional Medicine ................................................................................ 13
**CHAPTER II: Essential Botanical Defenders** .................... 17
  Echinacea: The Immune-Boosting Marvel ...................... 17
  Elderberry: Nature's Antiviral Elixir ................................... 20
  Garlic: A Potent Antiviral Herb .......................................... 22
  Andrographis: The King of Bitters ..................................... 24
**CHAPTER III: Cultivating and Harvesting Herbal Power** .. 27
  Growing Your Herbal Garden ........................................... 27
  Sustainable Harvesting Practices .................................... 32
  DIY Herbal Remedies at Home ........................................ 35
**CHAPTER IV: Integrating Botanical Defenders into Your Lifestyle** ................................................................................ 38
  Incorporating Herbal Teas for Daily Wellness ................ 38
  Cooking with Antiviral Herbs ............................................ 40
  Herbal Supplements: Choosing the Right Form ............ 43
**CHAPTER V: Herbal Antivirals and Modern Medicine** .... 46
  Complementary Approaches in Health .......................... 46
  Herb-Drug Interactions: What You Need to Know ........ 49

Collaborative Efforts for Immune Health ......................... 52

**CHAPTER VI: Case Studies and Success Stories** ............... 56

Personal Experiences with Herbal Antivirals ...................... 56

Clinical Studies and Research Findings ............................. 59

Inspiring Stories of Health Transformation ....................... 62

**CHAPTER VII: Navigating Challenges and Misconceptions** ................................................................................ 67

Common Myths About Herbal Antivirals ......................... 67

Overcoming Skepticism and Resistance ........................... 70

Addressing Safety Concerns .............................................. 74

**CHAPTER VIII: The Future of Herbal Antivirals** ................ 80

Emerging Trends in Herbal Medicine ................................ 80

Innovations in Botanical Research ..................................... 84

The Role of Botanical Defenders in Public Health ............ 90

**CHAPTER IX: Appendices** .................................................. 93

Recipes for Herbal Remedies ............................................. 93

Herbal Dosage Guidelines .................................................. 95

Glossary of Terms ............................................................... 98

**CHAPTER X: Resources and References** ......................... 102

Recommended Books and Publications .......................... 102

Websites and Organizations for Further Exploration ...... 105

References and Citations .................................................. 108

**CONCLUSION** ............................................................. **112**
Recap of Key Takeaways.................................................. 112
Empowering Readers to Embrace Herbal Antivirals........ 114
Looking Ahead: Your Journey with Botanical Defenders..118

# INTRODUCTION

"Botanical Defenders: Herbal Antivirals Unveiled - Harnessing Nature's Immune-Boosting Power" invites readers on an enlightening journey into herbal remedies, unlocking the potent potential of nature's botanical defenders. In an era where health and wellness have become paramount, this e-book is a comprehensive guide to understanding and harnessing the immune-boosting power of herbal antivirals.

As our world grapples with various viral threats, the need for effective and natural solutions has never been more critical. This e-book delves into the rich tapestry of botanicals, exploring their historical significance, traditional uses, and, most importantly, their scientifically proven antiviral properties. "Botanical Defenders" empowers readers to embrace a holistic approach to well-being by bridging the gap between ancient wisdom and modern research.

The e-book begins by laying a foundation of knowledge, offering insights into herbal medicine's historical and cultural contexts. It then seamlessly transitions into a detailed exploration of specific herbs renowned for their antiviral properties, providing in-depth information on their active compounds, mechanisms of action, and practical applications. Whether you are a seasoned herbal enthusiast or a newcomer seeking natural alternatives, this e-book caters to all levels of expertise.

"Botanical Defenders" doesn't merely stop at identifying these botanical heroes; it goes further by guiding readers on incorporating these herbal allies into their daily lives. From creating herbal infusions to crafting immune-boosting recipes, the e-book is a hands-on manual for those ready to embrace the healing power of nature.

In essence, "Botanical Defenders" emerges as a beacon of knowledge, demystifying herbal antivirals and empowering individuals to take charge of their well-being through the time-tested wisdom of botanicals. This e- book stands at the intersection of tradition and science, offering a holistic guide that inspires and equips readers to fortify their immune systems naturally.

# CHAPTER I

# The Foundations of Herbal Antivirals

### Historical Use of Herbs for Immune Support

The historical use of herbs for immune support weaves a rich tapestry of knowledge, traditions, and cultural practices spanning time. Herbalism, which provides a complex and all-encompassing method of preserving well-being, has been a vital part of human history, from ancient civilizations to indigenous populations. This section explores the historical foundations of herbal immune support, following the development of herbal treatments through various historical periods and cultural contexts.

Herbal knowledge was the mainstay of medical procedures in earlier societies. Herbs like thyme and garlic were used by the ancient Egyptians, who were known for their sophisticated medical understanding and in light of their possible immune-stimulating effects. Similarly, the old Indian medical system known as Ayurveda, which dates back more than 5,000 years, used herbs like ashwagandha, holy basil, and turmeric to strengthen the body's defenses. Herbs like echinacea, elderberry, and astragalus were recognized for their ability to support general health. They were included in the pharmacopeia of the Greco-Roman traditions, which included individuals such as Hippocrates and Galen.

Herbalism flourished in medieval Europe as monastic gardens turned into botanical knowledge banks. Medieval manuscripts referenced herbs such as chamomile, rosemary, and sage, which provide information on their potential immune-boosting properties. Herbalists such as Nicholas Culpeper promoted the availability of herbal medicines to the general public during the Renaissance, which saw a resurgence of interest in herbal medicine. The Doctrine of Signatures further impacted the usage of herbs based on their perceived similarity to particular body parts. This medieval herbalism-based idea added to the growing body of information about herbs.

For immunological support, indigenous civilizations worldwide have developed close bonds with native plant allies. For example, herbs like echinacea, goldenseal, and elderberry were used in Native American healing methods. Herbs like astragalus, ginseng, and medicinal For generations, traditional Chinese medicine has used mushrooms. To strengthen the body's vital energy and improve immunological function. Indigenous herbalism demonstrates a profound knowledge of local flora and its therapeutic applications for immune support across continents and climates.

During the Age of Exploration, herbalists witnessed the cross-continental flow of plant knowledge. Herbs like goldenseal and echinacea were carried from North America to Europe by the Columbian Exchange, while spices like cloves, cinnamon, and turmeric were brought from Asia to the West. This international trade enhanced herbal customs and increased the range of herbs that can be used to strengthen the immune system.

The development of allopathic medicine posed a threat to traditional herbal knowledge in the late 19th and early 20th centuries as industrialization spread. Still, herbalists such as Samuel Thomson and the eclectic doctors advocated for herbs to support immunological function. Movements against the mainstream during the 1960s and 1970s gave rise to a renewed interest in traditional healing techniques, which in turn gave rise to the rediscovery of herbalism.

Herbalism today reflects the historical usage of herbs to support the immune system. Native American tribes still regard echinacea highly as an immunity tonic. Elderberry has been used for its antiviral qualities by European herbalists for a long time. Astragalus and other traditional Chinese herbs are still used in contemporary herbal formulas to strengthen the immune system. The conventional understanding of herbal immune support provides direction for herbalists, naturopaths, and anyone looking for all-encompassing approaches to health.

The historical progression of herbal immune support highlights the long-standing connection between people and plants. Many cultures have contributed over millennia to our collective awareness of the potential of botanicals to strengthen the immune system. We are linked to the origins of herbal wisdom through the knowledge weaved by indigenous cultures, herbalists, and ancient healers, creating a tapestry that endures beyond time. The historical usage of herbs for immune support is a timeless source of inspiration, reminding us of the profound and enduring connection between humans and the botanical defenders that have withstood the test of time as we traverse the present and shape the future of herbalism.

## Science Behind Herbal Antiviral Properties

The intricate dance between plants and viruses has been a silent and ongoing battle throughout Earth's history. Recently, as scientific understanding has deepened, the spotlight has turned toward the remarkable antiviral properties exhibited by certain herbs. This section aims to disentangle the science underlying the antiviral qualities of herbal remedies by examining the defense mechanisms plants use against viral invaders and the potential applications of these defense mechanisms for human health.

A complex interplay of bioactive chemicals contained in plant cellular matrix is the fundamental mechanism underlying the antiviral properties of herbal remedies. Phytochemicals such as flavonoids, polyphenols, alkaloids, terpenes, and essential oils are some of the tools that plants use to fend off viral invasions. These substances have a variety of functions, including immune response modulation and interference with viral reproduction and entry into host cells. Interfering with the viral replication processes, which frequently results in inhibiting the enzymes required for the virus to replicate within host cells, is one of the fundamental strategies.

Herbs have antiviral properties beyond simply preventing viruses from replicating; they also strengthen the host's immune system. An essential component of herbal antiviral action is immunomodulation, which controls immunological responses to improve the body's capacity to identify and destroy viruses. Herbs such as echinacea, astragalus, and medicinal mushrooms activate T cells, natural killer cells, macrophages, and other immune system components, strengthening the body's defenses against viral invaders.

The virucidal qualities of several essential oils add even more depth to the field of herbal antivirals. Certain compounds found in essential oils, like phenols and terpenes, have direct antiviral activity that damages viral envelopes and structures. Three essential oils particularly noteworthy for their virucidal solid properties against viruses are tea tree, oregano, and eucalyptus. The way essential oils are used in aromatherapy, topical preparations, and environmental dispersion illustrates the variety of ways they support antiviral tactics.

Herbal antivirals interact delicately with the host's physiological systems outside the cellular and molecular battlefield. By reducing the conditions that encourage viral replication, their anti-inflammatory and antioxidant properties further amplify their antiviral benefits. Herbs that have a dual role in viral infections are turmeric, licorice root, and green tea. They directly reduce viral activity and lessen the collateral damage caused by the inflammatory reactions induced by viral infections.

Herbal antivirals are comprehensive and multidimensional due to the synergy of several bioactive components inside a single plant. The traditional usage of herbal preparations, which blend several plant allies to increase their combined efficacy, reflects this synergy. Ayurvedic and Traditional Chinese medicine, for example, take advantage of this synergy to formulate well-balanced remedies that fight viral infections and balance the patient's general constitution.

There has been a surge in scientific studies on herbal antivirals, offering factual data that supports conventional belief. Echinacea has been extensively studied for its antiviral effects, revealing its potential to modify immune responses and decrease viral replication. Native American tribes widely employ echinacea to enhance their immune systems. A mainstay of European herbal traditions, elderberry has demonstrated antiviral action against influenza viruses, mainly by blocking the entry of the viruses into host cells. Renowned in Traditional Chinese Medicine, astragalus has been investigated for its immunomodulatory properties, which suggest that it may strengthen antiviral defenses.

Herbal antiviral activities are complicated, and this flexibility to changing viral strains is part of their allure. Herbs frequently have a broad-spectrum action that hinders viruses from quickly developing resistance, unlike standard antiviral drugs that may struggle with resistance. This adaptogenic property, seen in plant allies such as astragalus and licorice root, guarantees that the allies stay potent against a wide range of viral threats.

It is critical to recognize this discipline's dynamic and ever-evolving nature as we continue to explore the scientific nuances of herbal antiviral activities. Even though scientific research offers insightful information, it is frequently a snapshot of the never-ending discovery process. Herbal antiviral research is complicated by the interaction between different populations of viruses and herbs, the impact of individual differences in sensitivity to herbs, and the synergy of herbal components.

Using natural antivirals in current medicine emphasizes how crucial it is to combine conventional knowledge with new scientific insights. While recognizing the potential for herbal therapies to supplement traditional techniques, the bridge between herbalism and mainstream medicine entails negotiating the subtleties of evidence-based practices. By combining the best aspects of both paradigms, this integration promotes a more patient-centered and holistic approach to healthcare that benefits those looking for all-encompassing wellness solutions.

Finally, the science underlying the antiviral qualities of herbs reveals a fascinating story of plant defenses against viral invaders. Herbs have a wide range of techniques to fight viruses, ranging from the complex mechanisms of inhibiting viral replication to regulating immune responses and the virucidal effects of essential oils. Conventional knowledge, supported by research, nevertheless directs the use of herbal antivirals in various cultural situations. The ability of herbal components to reduce inflammation and oxidative stress, as well as their adaptogenic and synergistic qualities, underpin herbs' diverse functions in promoting immunological health. The science of herbal antiviral properties invites us to investigate the relationship between human health and the wisdom of nature, where traditional knowledge and modern understanding converge in a dynamic dance of healing and discovery. Research advancements and the persistence of conventional knowledge foster this relationship.

## Differentiating Herbal Antivirals from Traditional Medicine

The distinction between herbal antivirals and traditional medicine unveils a complex and interconnected landscape where the roots of ancient healing practices entwine with the branches of modern scientific understanding. Promoting health and well-being is the shared goal of both fields, but they approach this goal differently, using different approaches and ideologies. By exploring the unique characteristics of each discipline and the potential for fruitful collaboration, this section seeks to elucidate the distinctions between conventional medicine and herbal antivirals.

Herbal antivirals use the innate qualities of plants to fight viral infections. They are based on the rich tapestry of botanical knowledge. This strategy uses various plant allies, each chosen for particular antiviral qualities. Strong antiviral properties can be found in plants, including echinacea, elderberry, astragalus, and essential oils. These plants can suppress viral growth, alter the immune system, and even directly damage viral components. Herbal antivirals combine the plants' bioactive components to create a complex and comprehensive defense against viral invaders. This is frequently why herbal antivirals work so well.

Conversely, traditional medicine represents a more comprehensive idea that includes various therapeutic modalities handed down through the years. Herbal medicines are included here, but alternative therapies include acupuncture, TCM, Ayurveda, and traditional indigenous healing practices. Conventional medicine frequently emphasizes a holistic approach, considering the connection between the mind, body, and spirit. A vital component of traditional medicine is the use of herbal remedies. Still, to address the underlying causes of sickness and restore balance, it also includes dietary recommendations, lifestyle changes, and spiritual components.

Differentiating herbal antivirals within the larger framework of traditional medicine emphasizes the particular emphasis on using plants that have been shown to possess antiviral qualities. Herbs are essential to conventional medicine, but the strategy goes beyond specific antiviral effects to include a holistic perspective on health and illness. Customized treatment plans, which consider the patient's particular constitution and circumstances in addition to the specific illness, are a common feature of traditional healing methods.

Herbal antivirals negotiate the boundary between custom and evidence-based medicine because they are based on conventional wisdom and modern scientific study. The discipline of herbal medicine is developing due to the renewed interest in herbalism and the scientific validation of traditional herbal knowledge. Studies conducted on plants such as echinacea, elderberry, and astragalus confirm their traditional applications and shed light on their modes of action. This synthesis of science and tradition highlights the versatility and applicability of herbal antivirals in the current medical environment.

While herbal medicines are included in traditional medicine, they also embrace holistic principles that recognize the interdependence of the individual with the environment, society, and the universe. Acupuncture, energy medicine, and mind-body therapies are among the practices essential to traditional healing systems across the globe. These techniques acknowledge the dynamic interplay of several elements influencing health and aim to restore harmony and balance. Conventional medicine's holistic approach aligns with the expanding understanding of the mind-body link and the influence of lifestyle on general health.

Traditional medicine strongly emphasizes prevention as the primary means of preserving health. The goal of dietary guidelines, seasonal practices, and lifestyle advice is to minimize the risk of sickness by laying the groundwork for optimal well-being. In traditional medicine, herbal medicines support the body's defenses, build resilience, and correct imbalances before they become illnesses. All of these things help to avoid disease.

A complete and integrative healthcare model could be created through cooperation between herbal antivirals and traditional medicine. Herbal antivirals can enhance the holistic principles of conventional medicine due to their unique antiviral and adaptogenic capabilities. Herbal antivirals can provide focused support for viral infections while addressing more general aspects of a person's health and lifestyle when incorporated into traditional therapeutic frameworks.

Working together, herbal antivirals and traditional medicine create opportunities for learning and cross-cultural interaction. A wide range of viewpoints on health and healing are provided by traditional healing systems, which are firmly anchored in regional ecosystems and cultural knowledge. Herbal antivirals must be incorporated into conventional frameworks with respect and cultural sensitivity, recognizing the distinctive contributions of each culture and creating a cooperative setting for sharing information and ideas.

Navigating the border between natural antivirals and conventional medication presents challenges. These difficulties include the possibility of herb-drug interactions, variances in diagnostic frameworks, and discrepancies in terminology. Open communication, multidisciplinary discussion, and a readiness to acknowledge the benefits of each strategy without discounting the other are necessary for effective collaboration. Bridging different worlds requires recognizing the need for both focused therapies and holistic viewpoints to promote health and well-being.

To sum up, distinguishing herbal antivirals from conventional medicine sheds light on the various healing modalities people have developed over the centuries. Herbal antivirals highlight the specificity and versatility of plant medicine with their targeted antiviral effects. With its more comprehensive range of therapeutic modalities, traditional medicine prioritizes a tailored and comprehensive approach to health. Herbal antivirals and conventional medicine work well together, and this could lead to a harmonious integration that combines the best aspects of both approaches to produce a holistic healthcare model. Setting out on a journey toward a more integrative, culturally rich, and holistic approach to health and well-being, we embrace the distinctive contributions of herbal antivirals and traditional medicine as we negotiate the complex web of healing traditions.

# CHAPTER II

# Essential Botanical Defenders

### Echinacea: The Immune-Boosting Marvel

In herbal Medicine, few plants evoke as much reverence and fascination as Echinacea. Coneflower, more often known, is a marvel of nature used for ages as a mainstay in herbalists' toolkits due to its many uses and immune-boosting qualities. This section explores the many facets of Echinacea, including its scientific basis for immune-boosting properties, historical origins, a variety of species and types, and valuable considerations for integrating this plant into regular wellness routines.

The history of Echinacea as a miracle for enhancing the immune system extends back through herbal history. Many Echinacea species, which are native to North America, have been essential to the medicinal practices of native peoples, especially the Plains Indians, who used it to treat various illnesses. Echinacea became known for its therapeutic powers as European settlers came across these traditions, and it eventually made its way into 19th-century eclectic medical practices. The plant's role in modern herbalism was cemented by its rise in 20th-century popularity fueled by the herbal renaissance.

Echinacea's reputation for boosting immunity is based on research that has attempted to identify the processes underlying its therapeutic benefits. Packed with bioactive substances like flavonoids, polysaccharides, and alkamides, Echinacea has a variety of effects on the immune system. Research has demonstrated that echinacea extracts can boost the synthesis of cytokines, which are helpful signaling molecules that coordinate the immune response and activate immune cells like macrophages. This plant's capacity to strengthen the body's defenses against different diseases is facilitated by its immunomodulatory action.

Knowing the various species and forms of Echinacea enhances its complexity as an immune-stimulating herb. Echinacea purpurea is arguably the most well-known and extensively researched species, possessing unique pink-purple blossoms. Echinacea angustifolia is historically significant to Native American tribes because of its conspicuous center cone and slender leaves. The striking pale pink petals and large cone of Echinacea pallida add to the variety of plants in the Echinacea genus. Every species has distinct phytochemical profiles impacting its medicinal uses and immune-suppressive properties.

Examining different preparations, doses, and possible interactions are important practical considerations when integrating Echinacea into wellness practices. Echinacea can be taken topically as salves or lotions or internally as teas, tinctures, and capsules. The particular health issue, the intended manner of administration, and personal preferences are frequently considered when selecting a preparation. The importance of dosage cannot be overstated; herbalists often recommend a calculated strategy known as "short-term, high-dose" to maximize the immune-stimulating benefits of Echinacea. On the other hand, appropriate use calls for considering specific medical issues, including allergies and drug combinations.

As Echinacea has become more well-known, the discussion about its suitability and effectiveness has also increased. The outcomes of clinical trials investigating if Echinacea can prevent or lessen the severity of upper respiratory infections have needed to be more consistent. While some studies point to a possible decrease in the length and intensity of symptoms, others show more subdued results. Variability in the preparation technique, individual response variations, and the particular Echinacea species employed can all impact the results of a study. Further investigation into the potential of

Echinacea to address other elements of immunological health, as well as its broader applicability in the domains of anti-inflammatory and antibacterial effects, is now underway.

Beyond its ability to strengthen the immune system, Echinacea encourages reflection on its significance in overall well-being. Plant energetics is a topic that herbalists discuss frequently, and Echinacea is no exception. Resilience and energy are attributes that Echinacea embodies with its bright blossoms and vigorous growth. Herbal traditions believe these energetic characteristics give people who work with the plant physical support and a sense of grit and empowerment. Growing and gathering Echinacea in a backyard garden or sustainably sourced preparations strengthens the bond between people and this plant ally.

The story of Echinacea is intricately linked to sustainable harvesting methods and ecological concerns. The herbal community has been discussing overharvesting and environmental loss due to increased demand for Echinacea products. Sustainable wildcrafting, horticulture initiatives, and ethical foraging methods aid echinacea population conservation. Herbalists support appropriate practices that guarantee the availability of Echinacea for future generations, acknowledging the significance of reciprocity.

To sum up, Echinacea represents an intriguing segment in the story of herbal Medicine that skillfully integrates traditional knowledge, scientific investigation, and real-world uses. Echinacea is a miracle of immunity-boosting plants that transcends its botanical identity to embody a holistic ally that appeals to those looking for resilience, vigor, and a connection to the natural world. The plant's transition from traditional herbal remedies to modern herbalism illustrates the continuing bond between people and the natural environment. Bright and versatile, Echinacea supports immunity and encourages further investigation into the relationships between science, tradition, and the continuous dance of health and well-being.

## Elderberry: Nature's Antiviral Elixir

The dark purple elderberry fruit (Sambucus nigra) has long been praised as a powerful natural cure for a wide range of illnesses, especially as an antiviral concoction. Elderberry has been used in traditional Medicine for ages, having its origins in herbal treatments and folk remedies from many civilizations. This section sheds light on elderberry's potential as a natural healing agent by examining its nutritional makeup, historical relevance, and scientific information regarding its antiviral effects.

Elderberry has been used extensively in herbal therapy for a long time. While Native Americans used its bark and leaves topically, ancient Egyptians employed it to cure burns. Elderberries were thought to offer anti-evil ghost qualities in European mythology. The 20th century saw a resurgence of interest in the medical usage of elderberries as scientists started looking into their possible health advantages.

The nutritional solid profile of elderberries is one of the main factors influencing their reputation as a medicinal fruit. Elderberries are a great source of fiber, antioxidants, and vitamin C, among other vital elements. These elements are essential for bolstering the immune system and advancing general health. The fruit's bright color and enhanced antioxidant qualities are attributed to the amount of flavonoids, specifically quercetin and anthocyanins.

Scholarly investigations have explored the antiviral properties of elderberry, emphasizing the fruit's ability to combat respiratory diseases, specifically the flu and the common cold. Researchers have found certain chemicals in elderberries to possess antiviral properties since they prevent viruses from replicating. Several clinical experiments have investigated the possibility of elderberry to lessen the length and intensity of viral infections; nevertheless, further investigation is required to draw firm findings.

Furthermore, elderberry has immune-stimulating qualities apart from antiviral ones. The fruit's anti-inflammatory and antioxidant properties have been researched because they assist the immune system. Extracts from elderberries have shown promise in regulating the immune system and strengthening the body's defenses against pathogens.

Elderberry has many promising qualities, but you should always approach it cautiously and be aware of potential adverse effects. Products containing elderberries may cause gastrointestinal distress or allergic responses in certain people. Additionally, using raw or unripe elderberries can be harmful because they contain cyanogenic glycosides. Adherence to appropriate preparation and consumption protocols is crucial in guaranteeing elderberry's secure and productive employment as a home medicine.

Elderberry syrups and supplements have become increasingly well-liked as over-the-counter antiviral choices in recent years, especially during flu seasons. But many different goods are on the market, and not all might live up to the hype. Consumers should use caution when choosing premium elderberry products and speak with medical professionals before adding them to their daily routines.

In summary, elderberry is a unique antiviral elixir generated from nature with a solid scientific basis and a rich historical heritage. Because of its high nutritional value and antiviral, anti-inflammatory, and antioxidant ingredients, elderberries can help bolster the immune system and mitigate the consequences of viral infections. Elderberry's full potential as a natural cure for general health and well-being can be unlocked if research in this area is conducted and used with a balanced and knowledgeable approach.

## Garlic: A Potent Antiviral Herb

Garlic (Allium sativum), a culinary staple with a rich history dating back thousands of years, has earned a formidable reputation as a flavor enhancer and a potent antiviral herb. Garlic has been praised for its therapeutic qualities throughout history and on many continents. It is essential to both conventional treatments and alternative medical approaches. This study delves into the various facets of garlic, looking at its chemical makeup, historical significance, and scientific backing for its potent antiviral properties.

Garlic has been used historically for both culinary and medicinal uses. Ancient Greek, Roman, Egyptian, and Chinese cultures were among those who understood the therapeutic use of garlic. It was widely used for everything from healing wounds and diseases to chasing away evil spirits. Garlic developed a reputation as a boon against the bubonic plague during the Middle Ages. These historical tales demonstrate the ingrained notion of garlic's therapeutic qualities, providing the groundwork for its ongoing application in various ethnic customs.

Garlic's complex chemical composition is thought to be responsible for its therapeutic properties. Sulfur-containing component allicin is believed to be one of the main bioactive ingredients behind garlic's antiviral properties. Crushed or diced garlic cloves release the enzyme alliinase, which causes allicin to develop. This molecule is a primary focus of scientific research on the therapeutic potential of garlic because it has shown antibacterial, antifungal, and antiviral effects in multiple laboratory experiments.

Research on the antiviral qualities of garlic has concentrated chiefly on how effective it is against respiratory illnesses like the flu and the common cold. Allicin has been demonstrated to inhibit viral replication, which may lessen the intensity and length of viral infections. Furthermore, garlic has immune-stimulating properties apart from its antiviral properties. It improves immune cell activity, increases the generation of white blood cells, and aids in the immune system's health.

Garlic has antiviral properties against various viral diseases, not just respiratory infections. Studies have examined the efficaciousness of garlic in combating the herpes simplex virus, HIV, and viral hepatitis. Although the outcomes of laboratory trials show promise, more research is necessary to translate these discoveries into practical applications. Much research is required to prove garlic is a dependable antiviral medication due to the intricacy of viral infections and individual diversity.

The medicinal properties of garlic extend beyond its immediate antiviral properties. It has antioxidant, anti-inflammatory, and heart-protective qualities. These characteristics support its all-encompassing effects on health and well-being. Garlic's potential as a flexible ally in preventing and managing various health disorders is highlighted by its links to decreasing inflammation, oxidative stress, and cardiovascular risk factors.

Garlic is a great food, but use should be done with caution, significantly when intensified or used as a supplement. Garlic can be uncomfortable for the stomach when consumed raw; too much of it might have adverse side effects. People allergic to garlic or have specific medical issues should also be cautious. As with any natural remedy, it is best to speak with medical professionals to ensure a safe and seamless integration into one's daily routine.

As a result of garlic's transformation from a common kitchen ingredient to a known antiviral plant, numerous supplements, and formulations containing garlic have been created. Popular products on the market include aged garlic extract, garlic oil, and vitamins made from garlic. However, there can be differences in the effectiveness and quality of these items, so buyers need to use caution when choosing trustworthy sources.

Compared to isolated components, the synergy of garlic's constituents in their natural condition may provide unique benefits.

In summary, garlic is a powerful herb with antiviral properties, a robust scientific basis, and a long history. Its complex chemical makeup, led by the ingredient allicin, highlights its wide range of therapeutic applications. Garlic is an excellent addition to any health promotion regimen because of its well-established immune-boosting, anti-inflammatory, and antioxidant qualities. However, research on its antiviral effectiveness is still ongoing. With more research, the full potential of garlic as a natural ally in the never-ending pursuit of wellness can be fully realized through a balanced and knowledgeable approach to incorporating it into one's lifestyle.

## Andrographis: The King of Bitters

Andrographis paniculata, commonly known as Andrographis, is a botanical marvel renowned for its bitter taste and potent medicinal properties. Andrographis, known as "The King of Bitters," has long been a mainstay in traditional medical systems, especially Ayurveda and traditional Chinese Medicine. This section explores the historical relevance, phytochemical makeup, and medicinal possibilities of Andrographis, illuminating the plant's varied uses as an herbal treatment.

Andrographis has a long history rooted in antiquated healing customs. Originating from South Asia, this herb is widely used in Ayurvedic Medicine and is referred to as "Kalmegh" or "King of Bitters." Traditional Chinese Medicine is called "Chuan Xin Lian." Its bitter flavor, which has earned it the nickname "King of Bitters," is frequently linked to its ability to treat various illnesses. Andrographis has been used historically to treat multiple ailments, from fevers and digestive issues to more complicated ailments like infections and immune-related diseases.

The phytochemical makeup of Andrographis is closely related to its medicinal potential. Its medical effects are mainly attributed to three bioactive components: andrographolides, neoandrographolides, and dehydroandrographolides. These substances, primarily present in the plant's leaves and stems, support the various pharmacological actions of Andrographis, such as its anti-inflammatory, antioxidant, antiviral, and immunomodulatory properties.

The antiviral effect of andrographis is one of its many qualities that has attracted much interest. Its effectiveness against several viruses, such as the human immunodeficiency virus (HIV), herpes simplex, and influenza, has been the subject of numerous investigations. Andrographolides demonstrate antiviral properties by preventing viruses from entering host cells and disrupting their replication ability. The encouraging results of studies conducted in vitro have generated interest in more clinical research to examine Andrographis's potential in treating viral infections.

Furthermore, Andrographis exhibits strong anti-inflammatory properties in addition to its antiviral properties. It suppresses pro-inflammatory cytokines to moderate the immune response, which makes it a good option for diseases with high levels of inflammation. This anti-inflammatory characteristic applies to viral disorders and long-term inflammatory ailments such as inflammatory bowel diseases and rheumatoid arthritis.

The immune-suppressive properties of andrographis aid in the plant's adaptogenic properties, which support the body's ability to withstand stress and preserve homeostasis. Its traditional usage in controlling and preventing infections is based on improving immunological function. Andrographis has demonstrated the capacity to activate immunological cells, including T lymphocytes and macrophages, strengthening the body's defense systems.

Although andrographis's bitter taste hinders its palatability, it is frequently regarded as a sign of its strength. Conventional medical systems explain the bitterness by saying it helps the body get clean and detoxified. It is thought that the bitter flavor increases the activity of digestive fluids, which improves nutrient absorption and digestion. Andrographis is well known in Ayurveda for its capacity to regulate the "Pitta" dosha, which is connected to digestion and metabolism.

It's essential to approach Andrographis with a nuanced awareness and respect for its potential adverse effects, just like any other herbal medicine. While bitterness is necessary for its medicinal properties, some people may find it difficult to bear. In certain instances, mild gastrointestinal problems like nausea and diarrhea have been seen. Furthermore, one should carefully evaluate the safety of Andrographis during pregnancy and lactation and seek medical advice before adopting it into one's routine.

Because of Andrographis's popularity, several formulations—such as supplements, tinctures, and teas—have been created. These commercially accessible goods provide different methods of utilizing the herb's acvantages. But Andrographis extracts' uniformity and quality can differ, highlighting the importance of purchasing goods from reliable suppliers.

In summary, Andrographis proves to be a powerful herbal treatment, deserving of its moniker "The King of Bitters," thanks to centuries of historical usage and contemporary scientific research. Its broad phytochemical profile highlights its flexibility, while its bitter taste indicates its powerful therapeutic capabilities. Andrographis has various health and wellbeing-promoting properties, including immunomodulation, antiviral, and anti-inflammatory actions. Andrographis is a botanical wonder whose full potential as a respected herbal ally can only be unlocked by a thoughtful and balanced approach to incorporating it into holistic health practices, even as research into its subtleties continues to reveal.

# CHAPTER III

# Cultivating and Harvesting Herbal Power

### Growing Your Herbal Garden

The allure of cultivating a personal herbal garden transcends mere aesthetics; it embodies a connection to nature, a journey into the world of healing plants, and a commitment to sustainable living. An herbal garden is becoming increasingly popular as people look for natural solutions to improve their well-being. This section offers insights into the transforming process of tending to and harvesting nature's medical abundance by examining the many facets of growing an herbal garden, from the therapeutic advantages of individual herbs to the practical issues of gardening techniques.

Taking up the task of cultivating your herbal garden might lead to an abundance of fascinating botanical discoveries. The first step is to choose the herbs based on your gardening tastes and health objectives. The choices are as varied as the advantages these herbs offer, ranging from the immune-boosting qualities of echinacea and the relaxing effects of chamomile and lavender to the powerful flexibility of mint. It is essential for successful growth to understand each herb's unique requirements, particularly water, sunlight, and soil composition.

Chamomile has long been valued for its relaxing qualities. It features delicate blossoms that resemble tiny daisies. When made into tea, the dried flowers provide a calming solution for tension and sleeplessness. Lavender, with its aromatic blooms, is a natural stress reliever and sleep aid, in addition to adding a beautiful perfume to your landscape. Meanwhile, the stimulating scent of mint leaves benefits respiratory and digestive health in addition to culinary uses. Echinacea is a striking accent throughout the cold and flu seasons, standing tall with its vivid purple blooms and supporting immune system function.

Growing an herbal garden is more than just planting; it's about establishing a balanced atmosphere that supports the health of the plants and the gardener. Comprehending the fundamentals of organic gardening, which eschews artificial pesticides and fertilizers, promotes an environmentally conscious and sustainable methodology. Accepting the interdependence of nature's design is embodied in companion planting, wherein certain herbs are put strategically to augment the growth and hardiness of other plants.

Based on conventional agricultural knowledge, companion planting maximizes available space while utilizing the beneficial interactions between various plants. For example, growing basil next to tomatoes enhances their flavor and growth, and marigolds can help ward against pests that could endanger the well-being of nearby plants. This all-encompassing gardening method creates a healthy ecosystem inside your herbal sanctuary by imitating the complex web of relationships in nature.

Choosing the suitable soil is essential to guaranteeing that herbs flourish to their full potential. Roots can grow in an environment that is well-draining and rich in organic debris. For individuals with limited space or less-than-ideal soil conditions, container gardening offers an alternative that provides flexibility in placement and maintenance. The particular requirements of each herb and the gardener's resources will determine whether to grow on open ground or in containers.

Proper watering techniques are essential to the upkeep of a robust herbal garden. Certain herbs, like lavender and rosemary, do better in drier soil; on the other hand, herbs like basil and mint do better in constantly damp soil. Root rot and dehydration can be avoided by knowing each herb's specific water needs and modifying watering regimens accordingly. Rainwater collected in barrels or other containers is a nutrient-rich, sustainable substitute for tap water that will further connect your herb garden with environmentally conscious practices.

One emerging guiding philosophy in herbal gardening is the idea of permaculture. Permaculture, which has its roots in sustainable design principles, attempts to replicate the diversity and resilience of natural systems by building self-sustaining ecosystems. With careful planning, an eye for natural patterns, and the development of symbiotic interactions between plants, insects, and other ecosystem components, you may incorporate permaculture ideas into your herbal garden.

Composting is a critical component of permaculture, which turns garden waste and leftover food into nutrient-rich soil amendments. As a result, less external fertilizer is required, microbial activity is encouraged, and soil fertility is improved. Culturing a wide variety of plants in one area, or polyculture adds to the general resilience and health of the garden. This method promotes a vibrant and balanced ecology while reducing the danger of diseases and pests.

Growing your herbal garden has advantages for mental, emotional, and physical health. Planting, tending, and harvesting in periodic cycles fosters a sense of interconnectedness with the natural world. The ability of gardening, sometimes known as "horticultural therapy," to alleviate stress, anxiety, and depression has been established. Taking care of plants, seeing them flourish, and enjoying the sensory delights of a garden, all contribute to a deep sense of peace and awareness.

With roots in ancient contemplative traditions, garden mindfulness invites people to engage with their gardens in the present moment. Every sensory experience, whether the soft rustle of leaves, the vivid colors of flowers, or the earthy scent following a downpour, adds to the meditation process. As a kind of active meditation, gardening helps practitioners escape the stresses of contemporary life and find comfort in the cycles of growth and decay in the natural world.

A well-maintained herb garden can serve as a source of culinary inspiration in addition to its medicinal properties. Fresh herbs from your garden add a palate of aromatic and tasty possibilities to home-cooked meals, enhancing their flavors. Freshly picking herbs right before using them in cooking maximizes their flavor and nutritional content. The culinary options are as varied as the herbs themselves, from the vibrant tones of cilantro in fresh salsas to the sturdiness of thyme in savory meals.

You can extend the year-round advantages of your herbal garden by drying, freezing, or making herbal infusions from the harvested plants. Herbal teas made from fresh herbs like lemon balm, peppermint, or chamomile provide a soothing drink with therapeutic properties. Herbal infusions such as lavender or rosemary allow for calming balms and energizing massage oils, among other natural skincare solutions.

Making tinctures, salves, and herbal extracts is part of using your garden to create herbal treatments. Herbs can be macerated in alcohol or oil to extract their medicinal ingredients, which can be used to make powerful treatments for various conditions. Homegrown herbal therapies have a wide range of applications. Two examples are echinacea tinctures for immune support and calendula-infused oil, which is well-known for its skin-healing effects.

Growing your herbal garden may provide specific problems like any other undertaking. Gardening inevitably involves pests, diseases, and unfavorable weather. Using integrated pest management strategies, like beneficial insect attraction and companion planting, helps balance the garden's ecosystem. Gaining the ability to recognize and handle everyday problems like powdery mildew and aphids enables gardeners to adjust and promote resilience in their herbal sanctuary.

Herbal gardening has educational benefits, including teaching people about plant life cycles and seasons. Certain herbs grow better in different seasons; knowing these trends will help you plan and maintain your garden. Certain herbs, like rosemary and basil, love the summer heat, while others, like cilantro and dill, are crops of the chilly season that thrive in the spring and fall. A plentiful and flourishing herbal garden is ensured by modifying planting dates and harvesting schedules by seasonal variations.

Herbal medicine transforms gardening into a path of self-awareness and empowerment. A deeper connection between gardener and plant results from an understanding of the energetics of herbs, from their tastes (sweet, bitter, spicy, etc.) to their affinities for specific organs or systems in the body. The herbalist's toolset is enhanced by the traditional idea of the "doctrine of signatures," which holds that a plant's look might reveal information about its potential medical applications.

As a result, gardening becomes a dynamic and ever-evolving activity that adapts to the seasons and the gardener's shifting demands. Creating, tending, and planting an herbal garden cultivates a sense of accountability and land care. Herbal gardening embodies the democratization of health and wellness by placing the means of healing directly in the hands of individuals, whether in a large backyard, on a balcony, or even in little pots on a windowsill.

Herbalism and sustainable living are becoming more popular, which aligns with a more significant cultural trend towards environmental awareness and holistic well-being. An herbal garden becomes a concrete and empowering way to embody these principles; it's a pledge to grow more natural cures and become less dependent on store-bought goods. This paradigm change also embraces wildcrafting, strengthening the link between herbalism and environmental care by allowing the ethical and sustainable collection of herbs from their natural environments.

Finally, cultivating your herbal garden is an undertaking that goes beyond horticulture and has a transformational and holistic quality. It explores the complex realm of therapeutic plants, a dedication to environmentally friendly living, and a celebration of the deep connection between people and the natural world. Cultivating an herbal garden is an invitation to begin a lifelong relationship with the healing abundance of the soil, from the therapeutic advantages of individual herbs to the practical considerations of gardening techniques.

## Sustainable Harvesting Practices

Sustainable harvesting practices are pivotal in maintaining the delicate equilibrium between meeting human needs and preserving the environment. Ecosystems are under tremendous strain due to the growing demand for resources brought on by the world's population growth. The practices used in harvesting, whether they be in agriculture, fishing, or the extraction of lumber, have a significant impact on the condition of our world. This section explores the various facets of sustainable harvesting, looking at the difficulties, inventions, and crucial requirements for a peaceful cohabitation between human activity and the environment.

One of the primary goals of sustainable harvesting is to ensure the perpetuation of ecosystems and their inherent biodiversity. Clear-cutting has long been a widespread technique in forestry, which results in habitat damage and deforestation. Reforestation, selective logging, and maintaining the ecosystem's potential for regeneration are all components of sustainable forestry methods. Comparably, overfishing in fisheries has become a major global issue, endangering both marine biodiversity and the means of subsistence for populations that depend on fishing. Sustainable fishing practices aim to slow down the depletion of fish supplies while promoting their regeneration. Examples of these practices include quotas, marine protected zones, and responsible aquaculture.

Since natural resources are frequently entwined with local people's cultural identities and economy, sustainable harvesting practices also significantly impact these communities. Indigenous groups, in particular, have a long history of demonstrating sustainable resource management techniques that put the long-term health of the ecosystem first. Integrating traditional knowledge with contemporary sustainable practices can foster a symbiotic relationship between communities and ecosystems. Furthermore, sustainable harvesting can help create green jobs that maintain economic stability without endangering the environment.

Many obstacles still exist despite the increased understanding of the significance of sustainable harvesting. Ecosystems are still being harmed by overfishing, illegal logging, and exploitative agricultural practices. Communities, scientists, and policymakers must work together to address these problems and implement sensible laws. Additionally, technology is essential to promoting sustainability. To verify that harvested goods adhere to sustainable criteria, tracking and tracing their origins using blockchain technology, artificial intelligence, and satellite monitoring is possible. Precision farming and agroforestry are examples of agricultural innovations that maximize yields while reducing their adverse environmental effects.

Certification programs like the Marine Stewardship Council (MSC) for fisheries and the Forest Stewardship Council (FSC) for forestry have grown in importance to encourage sustainable harvesting. Thanks to these certifications, customers may buy products confidently, knowing that they meet stringent environmental and social requirements. However, widespread adoption and adherence to the recommended principles are necessary for certification to be practical. There is also a discussion about how these certification methods need to be continuously improved and adjusted to take into account new scientific knowledge and meet new difficulties.

In addition, the growing effects of climate change emphasize how urgent it is to implement sustainable harvesting methods. The amount and quality of crops can be negatively impacted by typical harvesting cycles disrupted by temperature variations, precipitation patterns, and extreme weather. As a result, sustainable techniques need to be resilient and adaptable to a changing climate. Using ecological principles in agriculture, known as agroecology, provides a comprehensive strategy considering climate resiliency and sustainable production.

Customers have a big say in how sectors are steered toward sustainability. People add to the market for sustainable products by being knowledgeable consumers and endorsing products that bear official certifications. Campaigns for consumer education and awareness are essential in enabling people to make environmentally friendly decisions. In response, it is the duty of corporations and governments to be open and honest about the sourcing and production methods used in creating the goods they sell.

International cooperation is necessary to achieve sustainability because of the interconnectedness of ecosystems. Cooperative efforts are required to address transboundary challenges, including the illegal wildlife trade and the degradation of shared water resources. International agreements like the Sustainable Development Goals of the United Nations and the Convention on Biological Diversity offer structures for nations to collaborate in achieving shared environmental goals. Sharing best practices, technology, and knowledge can facilitate the global transition towards sustainable harvesting.

Sustainable harvesting methods are essential to the planet's ongoing health. A careful balance that considers the demands of both the present and the future generations is necessary due to the complex interactions between human activity and the environment. Assuring the resilience and vitality of ecosystems through adopting sustainability is not just a moral decision but also a prerequisite for industries ranging from forestry to aquaculture and agriculture. Sustainable harvesting is a ray of hope as we work through the difficulties presented by an expanding population and a shifting climate, providing a means for humans and the natural world to live in harmony.

## DIY Herbal Remedies at Home

In healthcare, the allure of DIY herbal remedies has become more popular as people look for natural alternatives to conventional medicine. Making herbal remedies at home has become famous for those who want to take charge of their health. It is based on ancient traditions and driven by a growing interest in holistic well-being. This section looks at the long history of herbal medicine, examines the advantages and disadvantages of making herbal treatments at home, and offers information on some popular herbs that can be used for complementary medicine.

The history of herbal therapy is rich, spanning thousands of years and several cultures. Herbal treatments have long been vital to healthcare systems worldwide, from Traditional Chinese Medicine to Ayurveda in India. Throughout history, civilizations have relied on the medicinal qualities of plants, such as herbs, as a reflection of their innate connection to the natural world. The recent interest in herbal medicines might be ascribed to the need for affordable and sustainable medical solutions.

The natural source of DIY herbal treatments is one of its main benefits. Many individuals are drawn to the idea of using herbs' many constituents, which can potentially have therapeutic effects, instead of the manufactured ingredients found in medications. Proponents contend that herbal medicines can enhance the body's natural healing abilities rather than only treating symptoms. This all-encompassing strategy fits nicely with a more significant movement toward lifestyle modifications and preventative treatment.

However, it's essential to know the possible hazards of using homemade herbal treatments. Herbal remedies have variable potencies and no set dosages, unlike pharmaceutical therapies. Because of this heterogeneity, safety, and efficacy issues exist since people might unintentionally take too much of the active ingredients. Moreover, there may be unexpected repercussions from combinations of conventional drugs and herbs, emphasizing the significance of making educated decisions and consulting medical professionals.

It's crucial for those starting in DIY herbalism to have an essential awareness of a few regularly used herbs. Well known for strengthening the immune system, echinacea is often used to prevent and treat colds. Similarly, ginger has become a household staple due to its anti-inflammatory and digestive properties. These herbs demonstrate the many uses of herbal treatments in everyday health, as do chamomile for calm and peppermint for soothing the digestive system.

Applying do-it-yourself herbal medicines goes beyond physical health, including emotional stability and mental well-being. Herbs like valerian root and lavender are well-liked options for reducing tension and encouraging sound sleep. The holistic approach of herbal medicine, which acknowledges the connection between the mind and body, is in line with the relaxing properties of these herbs.

Promoting a responsible and knowledgeable approach to do-it-yourself herbalism is essential as interest in herbal medicines develops. Education is a critical factor in enabling people to make knowledgeable decisions regarding their health. Reliable sources of information on herbs' characteristics, applications, and possible interactions can give enthusiasts the tools they need to traverse the complex field of herbal therapy successfully.

In summary, homemade herbal treatments offer an intriguing fusion of traditional knowledge and modern health techniques. Herbal medicine is seeing a comeback in popularity, indicative of a more significant cultural movement toward natural, holistic approaches to healing. The possible hazards associated with homemade herbal treatments highlight the need for caution and the value of making educated decisions in conjunction with medical professionals, even while the advantages of these cures are clear. A more sophisticated knowledge of regularly used herbs can open doors to a more customized and integrated approach to well-being as more people embrace the art of herbalism. Homemade herbal medicines can support a more comprehensive and long-lasting healthcare model in our dynamic world by fusing traditional knowledge with contemporary science.

# CHAPTER IV

# Integrating Botanical Defenders into Your Lifestyle

### Incorporating Herbal Teas for Daily Wellness

The ritualistic consumption of herbal teas has transcended cultural boundaries and historical epochs, weaving itself into the fabric of daily wellness practices. Drinking herbal teas is a long-standing custom rooted in the quest for mental, emotional, and physical well-being, and it has been practiced in ancient and modern nations. This section investigates the historical background of herbal teas, looks at the wide variety of plants used in these blends, and considers the possible health advantages of consuming herbal teas regularly.

Herbal tea has a rich history deeply ingrained in human society. Throughout history, societies have acknowledged the therapeutic qualities of diverse plants and utilized them by making herbal concoctions. Ancient tea ceremonies in China demonstrated the skill of making tea with medicinal herbs, fusing old customs with healing goals. Similarly, Indian Ayurveda promoted the use of herbal teas as a way to promote harmony and vigor by balancing the body's doshas. Herbal teas have long been prized for calming, healing, and improving human experience, from chamomile in ancient Egypt to mint in ancient Greece.

Herbal teas have become extremely popular today due to a growing consciousness of holistic well-being and a need for natural substitutes for traditional beverages. Thanks to the wide variety of available herbs, people can customize their selections for tea infusions according to their tastes and health objectives. Herbal teas are a fascinating addition to the daily routine because of their calming scent, cozy warmth, and possible health advantages.

Learning about different herbs and their unique qualities is vital to integrating herbal teas into everyday wellness. Renowned for its soothing properties, chamomile has long been used as a bedtime drink to encourage calmness and sound sleep. Peppermint is an energizing option at any time of day due to its cooling and digesting qualities. Prominent for its vivid hue and zesty taste, hibiscus is an excellent source of antioxidants that support general well-being. Because herbs are so adaptable, people can create a tea collection that explicitly addresses their requirements: immune system stimulation, digestive assistance, or stress reduction.

Herbal teas' popularity is mainly due to their numerous health advantages, which exceed their flavor profiles and sensory appeal. Renowned for strengthening the immune system, echinacea is frequently brewed as a prophylactic throughout the cold and flu seasons. Famous for its anti-inflammatory properties, ginger imparts warmth to drinks, facilitates digestion, and alleviates nausea. Herbal teas' all-encompassing strategy fits with a more considerable paradigm change in healthcare that emphasizes lifestyle interventions and preventative measures.

Certain herbs are essential for encouraging relaxation and stress alleviation regarding mental health and emotional well-being. Due to its relaxing scent, lavender is frequently added to teas to provide a mind-calming sensory experience. Renowned for its ability to elevate mood, lemon balm gives teas a zesty brightness and may also help reduce anxiety. Warm herbal tea served in a cup becomes a meditative act that provides a chance to unwind from the stresses of everyday life and for self-care.

People must approach incorporating herbal teas into everyday wellness with awareness and mindfulness as they navigate the confusing world of teas. Herbal teas are safe, yet several plants have contraindications for specific medical conditions or may interfere with pharmaceuticals. As such, seeking advice from medical experts and integrating herbal teas into a more comprehensive approach to health is crucial.

Herbal teas have a lot of cultural and historical value, and their possible health advantages make them more than just drinks. Herbal teas are now considered messengers of custom, healers, and conscious living. Herbal tea drinking, whether it's the energizing comfort of a chamomile blend before bed or the calming embrace of a peppermint tea in the morning, is a daily habit beyond simple hydration to promote overall well-being.

In summary, herbal teas for everyday health are a harmonious fusion of traditional knowledge with modern lifestyle options. Herbal tea's long history of use is evidence of its universal appeal over time and space. People discover a wealth of possible health advantages in addition to a world of flavors as they experiment with the various herbs that can be infused. People can develop a holistic approach to well-being by incorporating herbal teas into their daily routines, which will nourish their body, mind, and soul with each calming drink. Steeped in tradition and wellness, the art of consuming herbal tea inspires us to rediscover the profound relationship between nature and our quest for a more balanced, healthier lifestyle.

## Cooking with Antiviral Herbs

Lately, an increasing understanding of the significance of maintaining a robust immune system to combat various viruses and illnesses has grown. Using antiviral herbs in our regular food preparations is one fascinating approach that has drawn interest. Throughout history, traditional medicine has relied heavily on herbs, which are prized for their flavor and therapeutic qualities. This section explores the topic of "Cooking with Antiviral Herbs," looking at the scientific foundation, historical relevance, and real-world uses of these herbs in our meals.

Understanding the historical background of using antiviral herbs is crucial to appreciating their significance. For their therapeutic qualities, herbs have been valued throughout human history. Ancient cultures, including the Greeks, Romans, Chinese, and Egyptians, understood the medicinal properties of herbs and used them in their everyday routines. Due to these enduring traditions, herbal treatments have been passed down through the years. Herbs with antiviral properties have become popular because of the growing interest in using natural medicines in the modern world, where pharmaceuticals rule the healthcare scene.

The mechanisms behind the antiviral activities of several herbs are starting to be uncovered by scientific investigation. Strong antiviral properties can be found in many herbs' flavonoids, polyphenols, and essential oils. These bioactive substances stop viruses from spreading throughout the body by inhibiting viral reproduction. Two notable examples are oregano, which is high in carvacrol, and garlic, which contains allicin. These substances boost the immune system overall in addition to directly attacking viruses.

Thanks to its antiviral and immune-stimulating qualities, garlic has become a common ingredient in kitchens worldwide. Garlic's main ingredient, allicin, has been demonstrated to suppress viral replication and improve immune cell activity. Garlic, when added to food either raw or very gently cooked, can enhance flavor and nutrition. Comparably, carvacrol, a potent antiviral and antibacterial substance, is present in oregano, an aromatic herb frequently used in Mediterranean cooking. Not only can oregano add taste to salads, soups, and roasted vegetables, but it also strengthens the immune system.

There are many other antiviral herbs to try besides oregano and garlic. You can make a calming tea using echinacea, well-known for strengthening the immune system. Elderberries can be used in jams or syrups. They are known for their antiviral and anti-inflammatory qualities. Turmeric's primary component, curcumin, possesses powerful antiviral and anti-inflammatory properties. When carefully included in recipes, these herbs improve the taste experience and act as a natural protection against viral illnesses.

The practical application of cooking with antiviral herbs extends beyond mere supplementation; it involves a holistic approach to wellness. Including various spices and herbs in regular meals is essential to developing an immune-supportive and well-balanced diet. This strategy is best represented by the Mediterranean diet, which is well-known for its many health advantages and includes a variety of herbs, such as basil, thyme, and rosemary. Not only do these herbs improve the flavor profile of food, but they also benefit the general health of those who consume them.

It is critical to stress the value of moderation and balance in herbal therapy. Antiviral herbs provide many health advantages, but they should be used in addition to a balanced diet and a healthy lifestyle, not as a substitute. Strong immunity is based on a nutrient-rich diet, frequent exercise, and enough sleep. As a result, using antiviral herbs in cooking ought to be considered a seamless part of a more comprehensive strategy for overall health and well-being.

In conclusion, exploring "Cooking with Antiviral Herbs" reveals a fascinating intersection between culinary art and medicinal science. Incorporating antiviral herbs into our diets is a tasty and valuable way to strengthen our immune systems, drawing on centuries-old customs and bolstered by contemporary research. A wide range of flavors are available in the herb world to help create tasty and nutritious dishes, from echinacea and turmeric to garlic and oregano. Using these herbs in our cooking piques our interest in food and strengthens our body's defenses against viruses. The wisdom of the ancients, represented in these potent herbs, provides a roadmap for a balanced and nutritious approach to well-being as we negotiate the difficulties of modern health.

## Herbal Supplements: Choosing the Right Form

Within the rapidly growing field of health and well-being, herbal supplements have grown in popularity as more people look for natural remedies to enhance their well-being. But with so many different types of these supplements available, it begs an empowerment question: How does one pick the best herbal supplementation? This section investigates the benefits and drawbacks of several herbal supplement forms, such as capsules, tinctures, teas, and powders. People can maximize the ease and efficacy of their herbal supplementation by making educated judgments based on their understanding of the unique qualities of different forms.

One of the most popular and practical types of herbal supplements is capsules. Powdered herbs can be easily consumed and dosed precisely by encapsulating them in capsule form, so people with hectic schedules often choose them. Furthermore, capsules provide a discrete and tasteless substitute, resolving any concerns with palatability associated with other forms. It is imperative to consider the duration required for capsules to dissolve and discharge their contents within the gastrointestinal tract. Some contend that some herbs lose their effectiveness during the encapsulating process, which would restrict the active components' bioavailability. Despite this worry, capsules are still a sensible option for people who value ease of use and accurate dosage.

Conversely, tinctures are aqueous preparations of herbs that have been kept in glycerin or alcohol. This type of supplementation with herbs is highly valued because of its quick absorption, which enables the herb's active ingredients to enter the bloodstream more quickly. Since tinctures are simple to dilute in juice or water, they also offer dosage versatility. Tinctures' alcohol basis is a natural preservative, extending their shelf life. However, some people can find the alcohol concentration problematic, especially those who don't drink or have sensitive palates. Despite this, the liquid form of tinctures makes them a valuable and adaptable choice, particularly for people looking for quick absorption and adjustable dosages.

Herbal teas are a peaceful and calming way to include herbs into one's lifestyle. They are a timeless and pleasant tradition. Herbal tea is made by steeping fresh or dried herbs in hot water, allowing the flavors and health benefits of the herbs to permeate the drink. This method frequently requires a more extended steeping period than tinctures or capsules, but it offers a lovely ritual that many people find enjoyable. For those who value the ceremonial nature of making and drinking tea, herbal teas are especially advantageous. It's important to remember that some heat-sensitive chemicals in herbs may not be stable during the brewing process due to the heat. Still, herbal teas are well-liked and affordable, providing a tasty and refreshing way to take herbal supplements.

Herbal supplements in powder form, made from crushed herbs or plant parts, offer a flexible and adaptable choice. The powder form can be inventively added to various recipes, including soups, baked goods, and smoothies. Those who wish to include herbs subtly into their culinary ventures may find this flexibility in usage appealing. The powdered version can also be helpful for people who have trouble swallowing capsules or would rather stay away from tinctures that contain alcohol. With powders, it cannot be easy to measure exact dosages, which could result in consumption differences.

Moreover, some people may find the texture and flavor of some herbal powders unpleasant. Thus, creative methods to hide or improve these qualities are needed. Notwithstanding these drawbacks, powdered herbal supplements are popular for people looking for a flexible and gastronomically pleasing way to supplement with herbs.

In the end, selecting the best herbal supplement form requires carefully analyzing lifestyle choices, personal preferences, and health objectives. Herbal teas offer a reassuring ritual, tinctures offer quick absorption and flexibility, powdered supplements offer culinary variation, and capsules offer convenience and accurate dosage. Every form has unique benefits and cons, so people must consider these things while choosing the best choice. Furthermore, seeking advice from medical specialists or herbalists can be very helpful in ensuring that the form selected is in line with personal tastes and health needs. Making educated decisions is crucial when navigating the complex world of herbal supplements to maximize the advantages of natural cures while fitting in with one's preferences and way of life.

# CHAPTER V

# Herbal Antivirals and Modern Medicine

## Complementary Approaches in Health

In the evolving healthcare landscape, integrating complementary approaches has gained considerable attention as individuals seek holistic and personalized solutions to promote well-being. Complementary approaches provide a multidimensional approach to health and healing by encompassing many practices and therapies beyond traditional medicine. This section examines complementary and alternative medicine, which includes nutritional supplements, integrative medicine, mind-body therapies, and alternative therapies. By analyzing these methodologies' tenets, advantages, and difficulties, we understand their function in cultivating an all-encompassing and patient-focused approach to healthcare.

Complementary and alternative therapies are terms used to describe non-mainstream methods utilized in addition to or of traditional medical care. One such alternative treatment is acupuncture, a standard Chinese medical procedure that involves inserting tiny needles into predetermined body sites. The basic idea behind acupuncture is to harmonize the body's qi, or energy flow, to heal and relieve various conditions. Despite its antiquated beginnings, acupuncture has been more widely accepted in modern healthcare environments. Several studies have demonstrated its effectiveness in treating ailments like chronic pain, nausea, and even mental health issues.

Another group of complementary techniques that highlight the connection between physical and mental health is mind-body treatments. Activities that promote relaxation, stress reduction, and enhanced mental focus include yoga, meditation, and tai chi. Dr. Jon Kabat-Zinn created the mindfulness-based stress reduction (MBSR) program, which blends mindfulness meditation with yoga to improve resilience and manage stress. Studies show that Mindfulness-Based Stress Reduction (MBSR) can help with mental health enhancements, such as lowering anxiety and depressive symptoms. Including mind-body therapies in medical care reflects the expanding understanding of the relationship between the mind and body and the significance of treating both for general well-being.

Supplemental foods, such as vitamins, minerals, herbs, and other botanicals, are standard additional medicine. These supplements are frequently used to support particular health objectives or to close nutritional gaps, but they should not be used in place of a well-balanced diet. For example, omega-3 fatty acids from fish oil are well-known for their possible cardiovascular advantages, and people who don't get enough sun exposure may need to take vitamin D supplements. But there are differences in dietary supplements' effectiveness and safety, so it's essential to exercise caution—especially when handling large quantities or combining different supplements. When incorporating nutritional supplements into a health program, it's critical to consider each person's unique dietary requirements and seek advice from medical professionals.

The emerging field of integrative medicine presents a complete approach aimed at fusing evidence-based alternative therapies with the advantages of traditional medicine. This method, which takes a holistic approach rather than concentrating just on symptoms or illnesses, stresses the collaboration between patients and healthcare professionals. Various therapies, such as acupuncture, massage therapy, dietary counseling, and stress management, are frequently included in integrative medicine clinics. Integrative medicine seeks to improve patient satisfaction, maximize health outcomes, and enable people to actively participate in their well-being by fusing the finest aspects of complementary and conventional treatment.

Complementary techniques are becoming increasingly popular, although problems and disagreements still exist. Practices without strong scientific backing are frequently surrounded by skepticism, and integrating alternative medicines into traditional healthcare settings may encounter opposition. Furthermore, defining uniform benchmarks for efficacy is hampered by the heterogeneity in individual responses to different treatments. Another area of worry is the regulatory environment around dietary supplements. Different from the pharmaceutical industry, this sector is subject to different strict standards, which could result in variations in the quality and safety of products.

Promoting an evidence-based and patient-centered viewpoint is crucial when negotiating the world of complementary methods. Research is essential to determine the efficacy and safety of various strategies and to help people and healthcare professionals make educated decisions. Additionally, an integrative approach ensures that complementary therapies are used sparingly and with a complete understanding of potential risks and benefits by fostering open communication between patients and healthcare providers.

In summary, the adoption of complementary methods in health represents a paradigm change toward a more customized and comprehensive approach to well-being. Those looking to maximize their health can access various tools, including integrative medicine, nutritional supplements, alternative therapies, and mind-body interventions. While there are still issues and disagreements, complementary treatments can be responsibly and successfully incorporated into the more extensive healthcare system with the help of continuing research, well-informed decision-making, and honest communication between patients and healthcare professionals. The incorporation of complementary approaches is a tribute to the dynamic nature of health and our pursuit of all-encompassing solutions that foster resilience and vitality as we investigate the intersections of conventional wisdom and contemporary science.

## Herb-Drug Interactions: What You Need to Know

Individuals increasingly turn to botanical supplements to support their health as interest in herbal remedies grows. Herbal supplements have a long history of usage in traditional medicine, but there are some key things to keep in mind because of the possibility of interactions with prescription drugs. This section delves into the intricate realm of herb-drug interactions, illuminating the mechanisms at play, the variables that impact these interactions, and the importance of raising awareness among individuals and healthcare professionals.

Herb-drug interactions happen when the pharmacokinetics or pharmacodynamics of pharmaceutical medications interact with the chemicals found in herbs. Pharmacodynamics studies how pharmaceuticals affect the body, whereas pharmacokinetics studies how drugs are absorbed, distributed, metabolized, and eliminated inside the body. Comprehending these pathways is essential to understanding the potential effects of herbal substances on the safety and effectiveness of pharmaceutical treatments.

Herb-drug interactions are likely due to several variables. The bioavailability of pharmaceutical medications and natural substances is a critical factor. The percentage of a material that can be used therapeutically and reaches the bloodstream upon introduction into the body is referred to as bioavailability. A specific herb may impact a drug's bioavailability by changing its absorption, distribution, metabolism, or elimination. This could result in decreased efficacy or increased side effects.

The liver is the primary location of cytochrome P450 enzymes essential for drug metabolism. Certain herbs, including St. John's Wort, can stimulate these enzymes, which can hasten the breakdown of some medications and reduce their potency. On the other hand, several herbs can block these enzymes, which could slow down the metabolism of medicines and increase the likelihood of side effects by causing the drugs to accumulate in the body. Predicting and averting herb-drug interactions requires understanding how herbs interact with the enzymes in charge of drug metabolism.

Individual differences further influence the complexity of interactions between herbs and drugs in drug metabolism. Genetic variations can affect how drug-metabolizing enzymes function, resulting in variations in how people metabolize drugs. Drug metabolism can also be impacted by age, gender, and general health, which emphasizes the need for individualized approaches to treatment. The idea of pharmacogenomics, which focuses on customizing medication regimens according to a person's genetic composition, emphasizes how crucial it is to identify and take care of these unique variations.

Commonly used herbs that have shown the potential to interact with different drugs include ginkgo biloba, garlic, and ginger. Garlic, which has been linked to cardiovascular benefits, can increase the risk of bleeding when taken with blood-thinning drugs like warfarin. Often used for its anti-nausea effects, ginger may interact with anticoagulants and antiplatelet medications, thus increasing the risk of bleeding. Although ginkgo biloba is thought to improve cognitive performance, it may conflict with blood thinners and raise the possibility of bleeding incidents. These illustrations highlight how crucial it is to take herb-drug interactions into account when managing one's health on an autonomous basis and in clinical settings.

Physicians, pharmacists, and herbalists are among the healthcare practitioners who should know the importance of herb-drug interactions. Detailed medication histories are crucial in clinical settings where patients may use prescribed drugs in addition to herbal supplements. Healthcare providers must enquire about the usage of herbal supplements, keeping in mind that patients might only sometimes voluntarily divulge this information. A collaborative approach is fostered by open communication, which enables healthcare providers to provide advice on safe and efficient integrative methods.

As specialists in medications, pharmacists are essential in spotting and averting herb-drug interactions. They can provide information on the possible dangers of particular herb-drug combos, suggest suitable substitutes, and advise when and how much to take. In addition, pharmacists help patients become more educated decision-makers about their health and well-being through patient education.

With their knowledge of botanical medicine, herbalists are invaluable in advising people on how to safely and efficiently utilize herbs. Cooperative contact between herbalists and medical experts ensures a comprehensive approach to patient treatment. Herbalists can offer insightful information on the possible advantages and disadvantages of taking herbal supplements, assisting people in navigating the challenging field of integrative healthcare.

People also have a crucial role to play in protecting their health when taking prescription drugs and herbal supplements. It is essential to maintain open lines of communication with healthcare professionals so that they may offer individualized advice based on each patient's unique medical history and treatment plan. Before beginning a new herbal supplement regimen, people should seek expert counsel, educate themselves on potential herb-drug interactions, and diligently report all prescriptions and supplements they are taking.

To sum up, the intricate relationship between medications and herbs highlights the importance of having a thorough grasp of these interactions. These interactions include complicated and varied processes, including drug metabolism and enzyme function changes. Individual health conditions, genetic diversity, and bioavailability are some factors that influence how people react to combined herbal and pharmacological interventions. Healthcare professionals, such as doctors, pharmacists, herbalists, and people who actively participate in their healthcare decisions, share responsibility for managing herb-drug interactions. We can handle the complexity of herb-drug interactions and ensure the safe and successful incorporation of herbal supplements into healthcare regimens by working together, making informed decisions, and doing continuing research.

## Collaborative Efforts for Immune Health

In the ever-evolving landscape of health and wellness, the immune system is a formidable guardian, defending the body against many pathogens. Our comprehension of immune function is expanding, and with it comes the knowledge that promoting the best possible immune health calls for a multimodal and cooperative strategy. This section examines the various tactics and collaborative endeavors that support immunological health; these include dietary interventions, lifestyle factors, medical procedures, and the fusion of conventional and complementary methods. By analyzing the interrelationships among these components, we can understand how an integrative and cooperative viewpoint might strengthen the immune system and advance general health.

The basis of immunological health comprises lifestyle factors, which widely influence different aspects of well-being. An essential component of good health is enough sleep for immune system support. Immune response changes brought on by sleep deprivation have been related to an increased risk of infection. Regular exercise is another aspect of a person's lifestyle that supports immunological resilience. It has been demonstrated that exercise improves immunological surveillance by encouraging immune cell circulation and lowering inflammation. Sustaining a healthy body weight promotes immune health since obesity is linked to long-term inflammation and compromised immunological performance. Stress management is also critical because persistent stress can harm the immune system. Deep breathing exercises, yoga, and other mind-body techniques are excellent resources for reducing the adverse effects of stress and boosting immune function.

Nutritional interventions are crucial in maintaining immune health because they supply the fundamental components for a robust immunological response. A range of vitamins, minerals, and antioxidants can be obtained via a diversified, well-balanced diet high in fruits, vegetables, whole grains, and lean proteins. Specific vitamins, including zinc, vitamin D, and vitamin C, are involved explicitly in immunological function. Vitamin C aids in developing and operating immune cells and is present in citrus fruits and leafy greens. When exposed to sunshine, the skin produces vitamin D, which controls immune cell function and reduces inflammation. Meats, nuts, and legumes are rich sources of zinc, which is necessary for immune cell function and mucosal barrier preservation. The interdependent connection between immunological function and diet highlights the significance of consuming a diet that is rich in nutrients and well-rounded.

Preventive measures, immunizations, and tailored therapies are ways medical practices and interventions support immunological health. A vital component of public health, vaccinations encourage the immune system to identify and launch a defense against particular diseases. Vaccines have been crucial in the global control of infectious illnesses, thanks to cooperative efforts in research, development, and distribution. Furthermore, preventive actions, including routine physical examinations, screenings, and early identification of underlying medical disorders, support total immunological resilience. By treating underlying issues that may otherwise impair immune function, medical treatments for chronic diseases like diabetes and autoimmune disorders support the immune system's health.

A new level of collaboration is added to the efforts to promote immunological health by blending traditional and alternative approaches. Herbal treatments, dietary changes, and mind-body therapies are frequently used in conventional medical systems, such as Ayurveda, Traditional Chinese Medicine, and Indigenous healing techniques, to promote immunological balance. Adaptogenic herbs, such as astragalus and ashwagandha, are utilized in Traditional Chinese Medicine and Ayurveda, respectively, and are thought to boost immune system function and increase the body's ability to withstand stress. Likewise, incorporating complementary therapies such as energy healing, herbal supplements, and acupuncture enhances the comprehensive approach to immunological health. Integrative medicine's collaborative approach acknowledges the potential advantages of fusing ancient wisdom with contemporary scientific understanding, even though research on specific alternative approaches may continue.

Environmental factors, such as exposure to sunlight and outdoor surroundings, also influence the immune system's health. Spending time in nature has been linked to immune-boosting benefits, and sunlight is a natural source of vitamin D, which is necessary for immunological function. Beyond simple lifestyle choices, humans and the environment engage in a complex collaboration dance. By fostering a healthy and supportive ecosystem, sustainable activities that improve environmental health—like cutting pollution and protecting biodiversity—indirectly strengthen human immune systems.

Social networks and community involvement are essential components of teamwork for immunological health.

Overall well-being is significantly impacted by the social determinants of health, which include social support, economic stability, and access to healthcare. Communities that value chances for physical activity, wholesome food access, and health education foster an atmosphere that supports immunological resilience. Positive outcomes for mental and physical health, including immunological function, have been related to the sense of belonging and social support that communities provide. Community-based cooperation, whether via health education programs, support groups, or grassroots projects, enhances overall well-being and positively influences each person's immune system.

To sum up, the pursuit of immunological health involves a cooperative symphony of elements, each contributing in a distinct way to the body's defense systems. Lifestyle choices, dietary supplements, medical procedures, complementary and alternative therapies, environmental factors, and community involvement support the immune system's resilience and homeostasis. These interrelated components emphasize the value of a collaborative and holistic approach in which communities, healthcare providers, individuals, and the environment work together to build an ecosystem that supports immunological health. The cooperative efforts for immunological health become evident as we negotiate the complex dance between individual decisions, social context, and the larger environment. This shows how dynamic and intertwined well-being is.

# CHAPTER VI

# Case Studies and Success Stories

### Personal Experiences with Herbal Antivirals

Embarking on a journey towards holistic health often leads individuals to explore alternative and complementary approaches. Herbal antivirals present a compelling option in this vast field, utilizing the knowledge of traditional medicine and the therapeutic qualities of numerous plants. Experiences with herbal antivirals on a personal level frequently reveal a complex and unique approach to health based on the idea that nature offers a wide range of pharmacopeia to assist the body's natural healing capacity. This section explores personal stories that shed insight into people's experiences, difficulties, and victories when using herbal antivirals in their quest for well-being.

Many people are interested in herbal antivirals to boost immunity and prevent frequent viral infections. One person describes the annual custom of making elderberry tea in the winter, hoping the berries' alleged antiviral qualities would help prevent the flu. Compounds found in elderberries, which have long been prized in herbal traditions, are thought to suppress viral reproduction and alter immunological response. The decision made by an individual to incorporate elderberry into a daily regimen signifies a dedication to preventative healthcare as well as a link to ancestor wisdom that has been passed down through the ages.

Similarly, the well-known plant echinacea is frequently used in Western herbalism due to its immune-stimulating properties. A first-hand account describes taking echinacea tincture as soon as the cold symptoms appeared, and the person who did so reported feeling better and feeling better sooner. These examples support the historical usage of echinacea to treat respiratory infections and speak to the general sense that people are looking for alternative forms of self-care to complement traditional medical treatments.

The solid antibacterial qualities of garlic have made it a mainstay in the daily lives of people using herbal antivirals. Garlic has been touted for its ability to fight viruses and boost immune system performance, whether eaten raw, added to food, or taken as a supplement. Personal stories frequently center on using supplements containing garlic or including it in meals regularly during the flu and cold seasons. Garlic's intense flavor and perfume represent a proactive, all-natural approach to maintaining good health.

In addition to the well-known herbs such as garlic, echinacea, and elderberry, individual experiences extend into the domain of adaptogenic plants. Herbs with immune-modulating and stress-adapting qualities, such as ashwagandha and astragalus, have long been used in traditional Chinese and Ayurvedic medicine, respectively. People talk about how they have integrated adaptogens into their daily routines and attribute their sense of balance and resilience to these plant partners. The first-hand accounts emphasize the subtlety of herbalism, in which people customize their wellness regimens according to their requirements and reactions.

Although reports of successful personal experiences with herbal antivirals are common, difficulties and cautionary tales occasionally surface. One person reports getting upset after taking large amounts of potent herbal antibacterial oregano oil. This story serves as a reminder that although herbal medicines are natural, they may not be well-tolerated by everyone and can have unwanted effects. When adding herbal antivirals, one of the most important lessons learned is the value of starting with lower doses and paying attention to individual responses.

Furthermore, first-hand accounts highlight the need to procure herbs from reliable vendors. Since the strength and purity of the plant constituents are directly linked to the effectiveness of herbal treatments, quality and authenticity are essential. Storytelling frequently highlights the importance of getting herbs from reliable sources, whether buying items made from herbs or gathering plants straight from the wild. Considering this, it becomes essential to guarantee a happy and secure experience when using herbal antivirals.

The anecdotes highlight the cooperative aspect of herbalism when combined with more extensive medical procedures. People talk about their experiences seeking individualized advice on herbal protocols from herbalists, naturopaths, or integrative healthcare specialists. This cooperative method weaves a care fabric that celebrates the variety of instruments available to support health while acknowledging the importance of traditional and alternative viewpoints.

Furthermore, parental influences and cultural customs frequently collide with personal experiences. A person's experience with herbal antivirals may be influenced by cultural traditional medicine that uses certain plants or habits handed down from grandparents. These stories demonstrate a strong kinship with one's ancestry and an understanding that herbal knowledge endures throughout generations and transcends personal experiences.

In summary, individual experiences with herbal antivirals weave a complex picture of introspection, self-awareness, and resiliency. People navigate the realm of herbalism with a deep awareness of their bodies and a reverence for the healing potential of nature, whether they are using well-known cures like elderberry and garlic or the more complex world of adaptogens. Obstacles in the path highlight the importance of careful, informed research, while successful results build faith in the potency of herbal allies. These first-hand accounts add to the body of knowledge in herbalism by highlighting the unique and collaborative character of holistic health journeys. The stories people tell become strands in a larger story about rediscovering age-old traditions for a balanced and vibrant life and reestablishing a connection with nature as they continue incorporating herbs into their daily lives.

## Clinical Studies and Research Findings

In the vast healthcare landscape, the cornerstone of progress lies in rigorous scientific inquiry and investigation. Clinical trials and research findings form the foundation for all medical developments, treatment approaches, and health standards. The importance of clinical trials and research findings in influencing our knowledge of illnesses, treatment options, and public health campaigns is examined in this section. This investigation explores the dynamic relationship between scientific inquiry and better health outcomes, from the planning and execution of clinical trials to the conversion of research findings into practical applications.

Clinical investigations are essential for expanding our understanding of medicine since they are frequently carried out with human subjects in controlled environments. The goal of randomized controlled trials (RCTs), regarded as the gold standard in clinical research, is to assess the safety and effectiveness of therapies. Another popular kind of RCT is the placebo-controlled trial, which compares a treatment against a placebo to help researchers determine the precise effects of the treatment. Cohort, case-control, and observational studies offer complementary insights and valuable information on long-term outcomes, risk factors, and relationships. Because health research is multidimensional, many study designs enable scientists to address complex problems and find subtle links.

Reproducibility of results, statistical analysis, and study design robustness are critical for translating research findings into clinical practice. An important checkpoint is the peer-review procedure, in which specialists assess the caliber and validity of research before it is published. This thorough assessment guarantees that posted research adheres to accepted guidelines for methodology, science integrity, and ethical issues. The validity of scientific information is further reinforced by other researchers' reproducibility of study findings. Research findings provide building blocks for evidence-based medicine, assisting medical professionals in making well-informed decisions, as they are shared through conferences, peer- reviewed journals, and other venues.

Clinical trials are essential to the development and assessment of medications, medical devices, and other therapies in the field of therapeutics. For instance, drug studies go through phases, with Phase I am examining safety and dose and Phase II and III evaluating efficacy and adverse effects. Regulatory bodies like the U.S. FDA approve or reject medications based on the strength of these trials. FDA or EMA stands for Food and Drug Administration and European Medicines Agency. Novel therapeutics, from vaccines to cancer treatments, are introduced only after preclinical research and well-conducted clinical trials have been completed. The results of this research not only broaden the therapeutic alternatives available but also impact treatment protocols and standards of care.

Beyond treatments, clinical research plays a critical role in deciphering the intricacies of illnesses and the underlying processes that underlie them. Epidemiological studies offer important insights into disease prevalence, risk factors, and public health priorities by examining patterns and determinants of health and disease in communities. The genetic basis of diseases is revealed by genetic research, such as genome-wide association studies (GWAS), which informs targeted therapy and personalized medicine strategies. Studies that follow individuals over an extended period, known as longitudinal studies, aid in our comprehension of the natural history of illnesses and the variables affecting health outcomes. This research has a cumulative effect that goes beyond treating individual patients; it influences public health policy, preventative tactics, and the distribution of healthcare resources.

Clinical trials and research discoveries have been crucial in the context of infectious illnesses in helping to address global health emergencies. International collaboration among researchers is essential to developing vaccines, antiviral drugs, and public health initiatives. Clinical research is characterized by agility and cooperation. Vaccination clinical trials best demonstrate this, such as the ones carried out during the COVID-19 pandemic. The swift creation, examination, and implementation of vaccinations to combat newly developing infectious illnesses highlight the significance of a robust research framework and international collaboration. The public, healthcare professionals, and politicians use research findings to help them navigate the intricacies of pandemics and inform containment plans, vaccination programs, and public health messaging.

An emerging paradigm in clinical research, patient-centered outcomes research (PCOR), strongly emphasizes integrating patients' experiences, values, and viewpoints. This strategy acknowledges how critical it is to match research priorities to patients' treatment requirements and preferences. Including patients in all stages of the research process, from designing the study to disseminating the results, increases the study's relevance and practicality. PCOR encourages researchers and patients to work together, considering the many settings in which healthcare is provided and received. This methodology improves the caliber of research and allows people to engage in their healthcare choices actively.

Even with the numerous benefits that clinical studies offer, there are always obstacles to overcome to guarantee that research is inclusive and accessible. The generalizability of research findings may be limited by differences in research participation depending on criteria including gender, race, ethnicity, and socioeconomic position. Promoting diversity in research teams, creating studies that accurately reflect the demographics of the populations they are intended to serve, and including communities in the research process are all steps taken to address these inequities. Ensuring the integrity of clinical research is contingent upon ethical issues such as transparent reporting, informed consent, and protecting vulnerable people.

To sum up, the foundation of scientific investigation in medicine comprises clinical trials and research findings. Research has a wide range of effects on medical knowledge, from identifying illness causes to assessing therapeutic methods and developing public health policies. Clinical research is dynamic and ever-evolving, highlighted by its collaborative nature involving diverse teams and international interaction. Clinical research is critical in seeking better health outcomes and expanding medical knowledge, even as technology, methodology, and healthcare objectives change. We traverse the challenging landscape of healthcare via the prism of research findings, working toward a time when patient-centered care and evidence-based practice will come together to improve global health.

## Inspiring Stories of Health Transformation

In the tapestry of human experience, stories of health transformation weave a narrative of resilience, determination, and the indomitable spirit of individuals overcoming adversity to reclaim their well-being. These motivational stories speak to people of all backgrounds and highlight the common human desire for vitality and health. This section examines several stories that capture the life-changing experiences of people who, in the face of health issues, set out on journeys of recovery, introspection, and significant transformation.

A moving story comes from the field of chronic illness, where people struggle to manage complicated disorders that resist simple fixes. A rheumatoid arthritis patient describes in one narrative their initial feelings of anxiety and sorrow after learning they had the condition. When this person was told they might have a chronic illness that would change their life, they started a path that included complementary and mainstream medical therapies. This person had a significant transformation due to trial and error, lifestyle adjustments, and in-depth research into mind-body techniques like yoga and meditation. With time, managing symptoms evolved from a medical routine to a comprehensive way of life that encouraged resiliency and gave people the ability to deal with the difficulties of having a chronic illness.

Transformations related to well-being and weight loss are widespread in health narratives. Pursuing sustainable lifestyle modifications, self-image issues, and social pressures are common obstacles to reaching and maintaining a healthy weight. In one narrative, a person describes how losing weight gradually and sustainably—rather than using crash diets—was a life-changing experience. This person's journey required them to embrace a whole-foods-based diet, engage in regular physical activity, and deal with the emotional components of eating. The story emphasizes the value of changing one's perspective, practicing self-compassion, and realizing that improving one's mental and emotional well-being goes beyond improving one's physical look.

Intense tales of resiliency about mental health issues are remarkable because they highlight the transformational power of conquering psychological obstacles. One narrative describes a person's battle with anxiety and despair, describing how going to treatment, adopting mindfulness techniques, and creating coping mechanisms changed their life. The story emphasizes how important it is to provide mental health services, eradicate stigma, and promote understanding of the intricacies of emotional wellness. These tales demonstrate the transforming potential of self-awareness, resilience, and the realization that mental health is crucial to overall well-being.

The field of addiction and recovery offers an additional layer of complexity to the story of health change by presenting accounts of people who, in the face of substance abuse, find resilience and rejuvenation. In one story, the protagonist travels from the depths of addiction to a life of recovery characterized by self-reflection, sobriety, and a dedication to personal development. The main topic is persistence and the steadfast pursuit of a healthier, substance-free existence despite the individual's nonlinear route marked by setbacks and relapses. These accounts align with the broader narrative that portrays addiction as a chronic illness, highlighting the significance of continuous assistance, a supportive network, and a comprehensive approach to rehabilitation.

Physical fitness and athletics offer anecdotes of amazing health makeovers in which people overcome self-imposed constraints to accomplish astounding feats of fortitude, stamina, and strength. These tales include those who overcome setbacks to pursue athletic aspirations and others who, as they age, rediscover lifelong passions for exercise. The ability of movement, physical activity, and the pursuit of difficulties testify to the body's ability to adapt and grow. These stories encourage people of all ages to reevaluate their connection with exercise, seeing it as a source of happiness, self-determination, and long-term well-being rather than just a means to an end.

Narratives on the management of chronic diseases feature people overcoming the challenges posed by conditions like diabetes, hypertension, or autoimmune disorders. In one case, a person with type 2 diabetes is followed as they adopt lifestyle modifications to control their illness rather than giving up and living a life dependent on medications. Through dietary changes, consistent exercise, and continuous self-monitoring, this individual saw improvements in their general health and better blood sugar control. The story emphasizes how taking an active role in one's healthcare journey may empower oneself and how lifestyle modifications can significantly improve the results of chronic diseases.

Many times, the parenting path is a tale of health metamorphosis for both individuals and couples dealing with infertility issues and for those going through the significant psychological and physiological shifts that come with being pregnant. Tales of infertility include tenacity in the face of medical setbacks, mental fortitude in the face of setbacks, and the eventual success of conceiving and bringing a child into the world. Contrarily, pregnancy and postpartum narratives explore the life- changing experiences of adjusting to the mental and physical challenges of becoming a mother. These tales shed light on the human body's tenacity, the difficulties associated with reproductive health, and the transformational effect of welcoming a new life into the world.

Stories of cancer survivorship serve as moving testimonials to the life-changing experience of overcoming a terminal illness and emerging more robust and more determined than before. When given a cancer diagnosis, patients must negotiate the problematic side effects of the medication as well as the psychological cost of uncertainty. These stories highlight the significant benefits of resilience, support systems, and reassessing one's objectives in life when viewed through the perspective of survivorship. Cancer becomes a motivator for personal development, a return to one's fundamental principles, and a dedication to leading a purposeful, thankful life.

Together, these motivational tales of health transformation highlight the various human experiences when pursuing well-being. They emphasize the value of individualized approaches to health, considering that every person's path is different. Resilience, self-determination, and the understanding that a change in one's physical, mental, emotional, and even spiritual well-being are themes that run through all the stories. As these tales spread throughout communities, they act as rays of hope, providing consolation, direction, and motivation to those pursuing their journeys toward health and well-being. In the end, the mosaic of stories about health transformation adds to a larger story about human flourishing by serving as a constant reminder that, despite the ups and downs of life's obstacles, the possibility of revolutionary change is always there.

# CHAPTER VII

# Navigating Challenges and Misconceptions

## Common Myths About Herbal Antivirals

The world of herbal medicine has long been fascinating, with traditions rooted in ancient wisdom and many botanical remedies believed to offer health benefits. Herbal antivirals have gained prominence in this context due to their ability to treat viral infections. However, several myths and misconceptions have also gained traction alongside the sincere desire to use nature's healing powers to assist the immune system. This section aims to debunk widespread misconceptions about herbal antivirals by offering a balanced, fact-based analysis of their effectiveness, safety, and suitability for use in complementary and alternative medicine.

A common misconception is that herbal antivirals are a magic bullet that can treat any viral illness. Even though some herbs have shown antiviral effects in lab tests, it's essential to understand how complex viral infections can be and how different they might be when responding to herbal remedies. Not all viruses react to herbal remedies similarly, and the efficacy of herbal antivirals might differ depending on the particular virus, the patient's immune system, and the delivery method. Herbal antivirals should not be seen as a panacea; instead, they should be used with other holistic measures such as good cleanliness, immunization (if necessary), and teamwork with medical specialists to provide all-encompassing care.

Another common misconception is that herbal medicines are automatically safe because they are natural. It is untrue to say that they are risk-free because many herbs have been used for millennia without harming anyone. Bioactive components found in herbal compounds have the potential to trigger allergic reactions, interact with pharmaceuticals, or create adverse effects if taken in excess. In addition, there are hazards associated with contamination or misidentification of plants, and the quality of herbal products varies. Herbal antivirals should be used with the same prudence as pharmaceuticals; consult a certified healthcare provider and follow suggested dose guidelines.

The misconception that there is no scientific support for herbal medicines is also widely spread. In actuality, a growing corpus of studies is looking at the antiviral qualities of many plants. Research has examined the antiviral properties of astragalus, echinacea, elderberry, and garlic. Even if some studies point to encouraging outcomes, it's important to consider study design, sample size, and evidence quality when interpreting research. Furthermore, antiviral activity seen in lab tests does not necessarily correspond to clinical efficacy in people. Thorough clinical trials are required to confirm the effectiveness and safety of herbal antivirals in practical settings.

One well-known fallacy concerns the idea that more is better when it comes to herbal medicines—that is, higher dosages will result in greater effectiveness. The concept of dose-response connections and the possibility of adverse side effects at high doses are overlooked in this oversimplification. The dose-response curve of herbal compounds is generally bell-shaped, indicating an ideal dosage for therapeutic effects. Exceeding this dosage may not result in further benefits and may even raise the risk of adverse effects. It is essential to use herbal antivirals according to the recommended dosage, which reliable sources or medical professionals should direct to maximize benefits and minimize hazards.

The assumption that herbal goods are unregulated and can be used without any control is a continuation of the idea that herbal therapies cannot harm because they are "natural." This misconception is untrue; several nations have legal frameworks guaranteeing herbal products' efficacy, safety, and quality. The Food and Drug Administration (FDA) is authorized to regulate dietary supplements, including herbal products, in the United States by the Dietary Supplement Health and Education Act (DSHEA). However, customers must use discernment and select goods from reliable producers who follow quality guidelines, test their products for impurities, and give correct labeling.

One prevalent misperception is the idea that herbal antivirals should only be used on their own, without taking into account any possible interactions with prescription drugs. Drugs and herbal components may interact, either boosting or suppressing the effects of the drug and causing adverse side effects. For example, St. John's Wort has been shown to stimulate cytochrome P450 enzymes, which may impact how different drugs are metabolized and consequently lessen their efficacy. To fully evaluate any possible interactions and create safe and efficient treatment programs, patients must be able to discuss their usage of herbal antivirals with medical specialists freely.

The misconception that herbal antivirals act rapidly and relieve symptoms is a prevalent one, driven by the need for speedy fixes for medical issues. Although certain herbs can provide immediate relief from specific symptoms, their antiviral properties often take time to become apparent. Rather than offering quick fixes, herbal treatments usually gradually alter the immune system and antiviral pathways, promoting long-term resilience. When integrating herbal antivirals into treatment regimens, it's essential to be patient, consistent, and have reasonable expectations.

Finally, there is a common misconception that all herbal remedies with a "natural" label are the same in quality and effectiveness. The market for herbal supplements is broad and includes a range of products with different levels of strength, purity, and standardization. Techniques used in processing, harvesting, and cultivation can all impact the quality of herbal products. Customers should prioritize goods from reliable manufacturers to get the best outcomes; these should ideally be ones that follow Good Manufacturing Practices (GMP) and go through independent testing for purity and quality.

In summary, despite the potential of herbal antivirals as supplementary measures to enhance immune function, it's critical to dispel common misconceptions about them. A sophisticated comprehension of herbal treatments entails appreciating their possible advantages for personal health, being aware of their drawbacks, and using them with caution and knowledge. Herbal medicine research is still in its early stages, but combining evidence-based knowledge with conventional wisdom provides a well-rounded strategy for maximizing the therapeutic benefits of herbal antivirals while promoting holistic health.

## Overcoming Skepticism and Resistance

In the dynamic landscape of ideas and beliefs, skepticism and resistance are formidable barriers to accepting new concepts, innovations, or alternative approaches. When it comes to science, technology, medical, or social norms, resistance to change can hamper development and prevent the investigation of novel but possibly transformative avenues. This section explores the complex relationship between skepticism and resistance, examining the institutional, societal, and psychological aspects that influence these phenomena. It also looks at ways to overcome skepticism, cultivate open- mindedness, and balance critical thinking and the desire to venture into unfamiliar and unexplored areas.

Skepticism is the foundation of scientific investigation since it is based on a need for proof and a questioning mindset. But skepticism can also become more ingrained, impeding the acceptance of novel ideas with prejudices, predetermined beliefs, and a refusal to question conventional wisdom. Within the scientific community, opposition to new hypotheses or other explanations may take the form of defending the status quo. In this setting, overcoming skepticism necessitates a careful balancing act between upholding the strict criteria of scientific proof and cultivating an atmosphere promoting the investigation of non-conventional theories. From the heliocentric model to the idea of evolution, the history of scientific revolutions demonstrates the transformational power of questioning established wisdom and dispelling deep-seated doubt.

From a psychological perspective, skepticism frequently results from a fear of the unknown or cognitive dissonance brought on by information that challenges preconceived notions. People could cling to well-known concepts to preserve their sense of stability and security. Individuals can overcome skepticism by developing an open-minded perspective, embracing inquiry, and realizing that reevaluating and reviewing one's ideas is frequently necessary for intellectual growth. Overcoming personal skepticism necessitates humility, an openness to learning, and an awareness that intellectual development is an ongoing process.

Social and cultural variables play a significant role in the resistance and general mistrust of the group. Communities' worldviews are shaped by cultural norms, customs, and shared ideologies, which can lead to opposition to concepts that go against the status quo. A fear of social rejection or identity loss can further cement skepticism within organizations. To overcome cultural skepticism, one must encourage communication, advance learning, and emphasize how novel concepts align with fundamental principles. A more inclusive and adaptable societal mindset can be facilitated by initiatives that balance tradition and innovation, highlighting the continuity of cultural identity while welcoming new viewpoints.

Adopting innovative methods can face significant obstacles due to institutional inertia, which can occur in academic institutions, healthcare systems, or other organizational structures. Hierarchy, established rules, and deeply ingrained traditions can foster resistance to change. Overcoming institutional skepticism requires a dedication to promoting an innovative culture, offering rewards for investigating alternate approaches, and removing obstacles that prevent the acceptance of novel concepts. Organizational cultures can move away from skepticism and toward a more dynamic and responsive ethos when leaders foster various thoughts, value innovation, and reward flexibility.

Overcoming skepticism is especially important in medicine because it directly affects patient care and well-being. The medical community is skeptical of complementary and alternative therapies, and some practitioners are hesitant to deviate from evidence-based practices. It takes a sophisticated grasp of the advantages and disadvantages of complementary therapies and traditional medicine to bridge the gap between them effectively. Integrative medicine models provide a cooperative, patient-centered approach that tackles skepticism and the possible advantages of holistic care. These models integrate evidence-based conventional therapies with specific alternative techniques. Research examining the synergies between traditional and alternative therapies and continual education and open communication are necessary to overcome reluctance within the medical profession.

Technological innovations are also often met with skepticism, particularly when they extend the bounds of what was previously believed to be feasible. Emerging technologies like genetic editing, artificial intelligence, and quantum computing may encounter opposition from people worried about the long-term effects, employment displacement, or ethical issues. Robust ethical frameworks, open communication about possible dangers and rewards, and a dedication to inclusive and participatory decision-making are all necessary to overcome technological skepticism. A more knowledgeable and accommodating society attitude toward emerging technologies can be achieved by public participation, education, and cooperative efforts among technologists, ethicists, and legislators.

Effective communication becomes essential for promoting acceptance and understanding when faced with opposition and doubt. Communicators must struggle between addressing concerns, offering solid arguments, and admitting that new concepts or methods have inherent complications. Abstract ideas can be humanized and made more approachable and understandable by storytelling, anecdotes, and relevant examples. Developing communication bridges requires empathy, active listening, and a sincere attempt to comprehend the viewpoints and worries of doubters. Overcoming resistance and establishing an atmosphere favorable to change need the creation of forums for polite conversation where opposing viewpoints are acknowledged and considered.

Since education equips people with knowledge and critical thinking abilities, it is essential for overcoming skepticism. In addition to providing knowledge, educational programs should foster intellectual curiosity, flexibility, and a readiness to challenge presumptions. A culture of open-minded inquiry can be promoted by including many viewpoints in academic curricula, encouraging interdisciplinary learning, and exposing students to various ideas. Adopting lifelong learning as a fundamental principle makes society more adaptable and robust, making it less susceptible to deeply ingrained skepticism.

Whether in business, governance, healthcare, or scientific research, leadership is essential in forming organizational cultures and perspectives on innovation. Leaders who promote experimentation, risk-taking, and rewarding learning from mistakes foster cultures where skepticism is viewed as a chance for improvement rather than a barrier. Breaking down barriers to change, inclusive leadership that supports a variety of viewpoints, opinions, and experiences promotes a more collaborative and receptive environment.

Individual skepticism can be addressed using psychological procedures such as mindfulness exercises, cognitive-behavioral approaches, and story therapy. These methods seek to dispel anxiety about the unknown, detect and combat cognitive biases, and foster cognitive flexibility. An open and flexible mindset can be promoted by encouraging people to investigate the underlying assumptions underlying their skepticism and offering resources for perspective-reframing.

Cultural change is a complex but necessary process that entails questioning deeply held beliefs and changing how society views creativity and uniqueness. A culture change can be facilitated by grassroots movements, cultural influencers, and programs that honor a variety of opinions. Accepting cultural narratives that emphasize the advantages of curiosity, flexibility, and an openness to learning helps create an atmosphere in which skepticism is seen as an opportunity for development rather than a danger.

In summary, overcoming opposition and doubt necessitates a complex strategy that considers institutional, societal, and psychological factors. Progress and human advancement are contingent upon the capacity to negotiate skepticism, whether in science, health, technology, or societal norms. Societies can overcome the constraints of skepticism and bring about revolutionary change by promoting open-mindedness, accepting multiple viewpoints, and creating conditions that encourage innovation. Overcoming skepticism is a lifelong effort that requires curiosity, humility, and a dedication to fostering an environment that promotes knowledge and innovation.

## Addressing Safety Concerns

Safety concerns permeate every facet of human existence, from the food we consume to the medications we take, the technologies we adopt, and the environments we inhabit. The quest for development frequently collides with concerns about safety in an era of unparalleled scientific and technical advancements, forcing people, communities, and policymakers to consider the advantages and disadvantages of novel solutions. This section examines the complexity of safety concerns by examining the difficulties in identifying, evaluating, and conveying hazards in various contexts. In technology, medicine, and environmental sustainability, among others, the need to address safety concerns emphasizes the fine line that must be drawn between innovation and the preservation of human welfare.

Safety considerations are fundamental to the development, testing, and delivery of drugs and medical interventions in the field of medicine. Careful testing in preclinical and clinical settings is necessary for the rigorous drug development process to evaluate safety and efficacy. Unexpected side effects, however, can still surface even after thorough testing. Continuous surveillance, comprehensive post-marketing monitoring, and open communication between the public, regulatory bodies, and healthcare professionals are required to address safety concerns in medicine. The introduction of pharmacovigilance systems, which methodically gather, examine, and share data regarding drug safety, is a prime example of the dedication to ongoing assessment and development.

One of the main issues with medical safety is vaccine safety, particularly in light of international immunization programs. Careful inspection is necessary to guarantee the effectiveness and safety of vaccinations against infectious illnesses during production and distribution. The public's trust in immunization programs depends on open and honest disclosure about possible side effects, stringent testing protocols, and continuous observation of infrequent adverse events. The necessity for evidence-based decision-making, precise communication methods, and cooperation between regulatory agencies and healthcare providers is highlighted by the delicate balance between immunization's possible dangers and benefits.

Extra safety precautions exist when using medical devices, such as implants and diagnostic gadgets. Strict testing, governmental supervision, and post-market surveillance are required to guarantee these products' dependability, robustness, and safety. Medical device safety issues necessitate a proactive strategy that foresees possible dangers and considers user input to improve features and designs. The convergence of technology and healthcare, as seen by the growth of wearables and telemedicine, adds additional safety considerations that necessitate constant evaluation and modification.

Beyond the healthcare industry, the quick development of technology in other fields raises security issues ranging from personal privacy to the welfare of society as a whole. The widespread application of machine learning and artificial intelligence (AI) raises concerns about the adverse effects of automated decision-making, biases in data sets, and the morality of using algorithms. Technology-related safety issues necessitate interdisciplinary cooperation between ethicists, legislators, technologists, and the general public. Creating frameworks that put fairness, accountability, and transparency first becomes crucial to negotiating the ethical implications of emerging technology.

Cybersecurity is a critical safety concern in an increasingly linked world, where hazards to individuals, corporations, and governments come from identity theft, data breaches, and cyberattacks. Information and communication systems are rapidly becoming digital, necessitating ongoing security measure adaption, the creation of robust encryption technologies, and international collaboration to combat cyber attacks. Digital infrastructure security affects personal privacy and the reliability of crucial infrastructure, financial institutions, and national security.

Concerns over pollution, climate change, and resource depletion highlight the complex interrelationship between human activity and the state of the planet in the context of environmental safety. An all-encompassing strategy that includes conservation initiatives, sustainable behaviors, and policy interventions is required to address safety concerns in the environmental domain. Global efforts to lessen the effects of human activity on the environment must prioritize switching to renewable energy sources, waste reduction programs, and biodiversity preservation. In this context, safety refers to maintaining ecosystems and the delicate balance of Earth's natural processes in addition to the immediate well-being of humans.

Occupational safety and health at work become increasingly important factors, especially when work settings change and become more diverse. To guarantee employees' physical and mental health, safety procedures must be followed, sufficient training must be given, and issues pertaining to ergonomic design and psychosocial aspects must be addressed. With the rise of remote work, there are no additional safety concerns to be aware of, such as the requirement for cybersecurity safeguards, ways to avoid digital burnout, and methods to preserve a positive work-life balance.

Regarding transportation, safety concerns range from the security of individual vehicles to the layout of infrastructure and systems. The automotive industry's dedication to creating safer automobiles, integrating cutting-edge driver assistance systems, and investigating autonomous technologies indicates its continuous efforts to improve safety. Reducing the dangers of traffic accidents, air pollution, and congestion largely depends on the architecture of transportation networks and urban planning. To develop safe and sustainable mobility solutions, industry, governments, and urban planners must work together at the crossroads of safety, technology, and transportation.

Concerns about consumer product safety include everything from the safety of toys, household goods, and recreational equipment to the caliber of food and drink. Regulatory bodies are pivotal in setting safety guidelines, carrying out examinations, and releasing recalls as required. Protecting people from potential injury related to consumer goods is facilitated by manufacturer adherence to safety laws, consumer education, and labeling requirements.

In a pandemic or other public health emergency, addressing safety concerns requires rapid response procedures, international cooperation, and the establishment of solid healthcare infrastructures. The current COVID-19 epidemic is an example of how difficult it is to manage safety issues worldwide. Campaigns for vaccination, public health measures, and communication tactics are all crucial parts of the global effort to lessen the virus's effects and safeguard people.

One of the most important aspects of resolving safety problems in various fields is properly communicating safety information. Communication tactics that are open, approachable, and mindful of cultural differences support informed decision-making and build public confidence. When it comes to spreading truthful information, busting myths, and promoting responsible behavior, the roles of the media, social influencers, and community leaders become vital. Governments, medical experts, scientists, and communicators must work together to create narratives emphasizing safety, refuting false information, and giving people the power to make decisions that will improve their well-being.

Handling safety issues is a complex and diverse undertaking that crosses several fields, including technology, medicine, the environment, and more. The quest for advancement and novelty inevitably entails managing possible hazards, requiring a dedication to stringent examination, continuous observation, and open correspondence. The careful balancing act between promoting progress and protecting people's health calls for interdisciplinary cooperation, safety-focused regulatory frameworks, and a dedication to moral behavior. Individuals, communities, and policymakers all have a crucial role in creating a future where innovation and well-being coexist peacefully in the complicated fabric of safety considerations.

# CHAPTER VIII

# The Future of Herbal Antivirals

## Emerging Trends in Herbal Medicine

Herbal Herbal medicine, rooted in ancient traditions and practices, has experienced a resurgence in interest and exploration in recent years. Herbal medicine is coming into its own as communities look for more sustainable and holistic ways to healthcare, with new emerging trends combining ancient knowledge with cutting-edge research. This section explores the nexus between traditional wisdom, new technology, and modern healthcare demands as it looks at the developing trends in herbal medicine. A sophisticated awareness of herbal medicine's possible advantages, difficulties, and future directions is reflected in the changing landscape, which ranges from customized herbal formulations to the incorporation of herbal medicine into traditional healthcare.

Personalized herbal formulations based on a patient's unique health needs are a popular trend in herbal treatment. Customized approaches are becoming increasingly popular among practitioners as they realize that distinct health profiles, lifestyle choices, and genetics can all affect an individual's response to herbal medicines. This movement is in line with the more general personalized medicine paradigm, which tailors medical interventions to the unique needs of individual patients. Precision herbal treatment is becoming increasingly popular, partly due to developments in genetic research and investigation of personal variances in reaction to herbal substances. By incorporating technology like metabolomics and genetic testing, practitioners can find the best herbal formulations, doses, and delivery systems for improved therapeutic results.

Another developing area in herbal medicine is the study of herbal mixtures and plant synergies. The synergistic effects of mixing various plants are widely utilized in traditional herbal systems to improve medicinal efficacy and reduce potential adverse effects. The contemporary study explores the complex interrelationships among herbal chemicals to comprehend how combining particular herbs may produce synergies that exceed the impact of individual constituents. This concept encourages the creation of comprehensive formulations that use the complementary activities of many plant components, moving beyond single-herb methods. The study of herbal combinations is in line with the holistic ideas of herbal therapy, which hold that the whole of a plant is greater than the sum of its parts.

Standardization and quality control are essential factors in the new developments in herbal medicine. Making sure botanical preparations are consistent and safe is a significant challenge as demand for herbal products rises. Regulatory authorities and industry standards are changing to address concerns about adulteration, mislabeling, and variances in the quality of herbal products. Advanced analytical methods allow for identifying and measuring particular substances in herbal products, such as DNA barcoding and high-performance liquid chromatography (HPLC). Herbal extracts are standardized for their bioactive components, guaranteeing they remain high-quality and potent. These advancements help solidify herbal medicine's position as a dependable and repeatable treatment.

A revolutionary movement toward a more inclusive and team-based approach to patient care is incorporating herbal medicine into traditional healthcare. Global healthcare systems promote integrative or complementary medicine by realizing the benefits of herbal and conventional therapies. A growing amount of scientific research is demonstrating the effectiveness and safety of some herbal remedies, which is driving this trend. Herbalists, naturopathic doctors, and conventional healthcare professionals are working together to provide patients with all-encompassing, customized care that combines the best elements of traditional and modern medicine. According to integrative healthcare models, herbal medicine has a place in chronic illness management, preventive care, and general well-being.

As the need for evidence-based herbal treatment grows, the fields of clinical research and randomized controlled trials (RCTs) are becoming increasingly important. Herbal medicine is based on traditional knowledge, but thorough scientific research adds to its credibility, guides clinical practice, and expands our body of medical knowledge. The safety, effectiveness, and mechanisms of action of herbal therapies are clarified through the planning and implementation of carefully monitored research. This tendency is consistent with evidence-based medicine, which bases patient care decisions on the best available scientific data. The increasing amount of research raises the legitimacy of herbal therapy and makes it easier for patients and healthcare professionals to have educated conversations.

As environmental consciousness grows in importance worldwide, there is a change in herbal therapy toward sustainable and ethical approaches. Sustainable gardening techniques are replacing the traditional practice of wildcrafting, which involves gathering herbs from their native environments. Culturing medicinal plants in regulated settings, like organic farms or botanical gardens, minimizes the disturbance of natural ecosystems and guarantees a sustainable supply. Beyond farming, ethical issues involve biodiversity preservation, fair trade methods, and community assistance. The broader movement toward ecologically conscious healthcare and responsible resource management aligns with the trend toward sustainable and ethical herbal practices.

A significant trend that is beginning to take shape is the investigation of herbal medicine about mental health and well-being. Ayurveda and Traditional Chinese Medicine (TCM) are two examples of traditional medical systems that have long acknowledged the connection between psychological and physical health. Current studies are revealing the psychotropic properties of several herbal substances and their possible uses in the treatment of depression, anxiety, stress, and cognitive impairment. Herbs, known as adaptogens, which aid in the body's adjustment to stress, are becoming increasingly well-known for their capacity to foster resilience and mental health. Herbal medicine's incorporation into mental health treatment complements traditional methods, providing a comprehensive understanding of mental and emotional equilibrium variables.

Advances in herbal delivery methods are revolutionizing the administration of herbal medications, improving patient compliance, convenience, and effectiveness. Novel formulations, including herbal capsules, pills, and standardized extracts, are being added to traditional means of preparation like teas, tinctures, and decoctions. Developing targeted delivery systems aims to maximize therapeutic benefits and increase bioavailability. One example of this is encapsulating herbal components in nanoparticles. These developments help modernize herbal therapy, increasing its accessibility and attractiveness to people who are used to traditional pharmaceutical forms.

Another trend in herbal medicine is the exchange of herbal knowledge across countries and traditions and global cooperation. Herbalists, researchers, and healthcare professionals from various backgrounds exchange knowledge, experiences, and research findings as communication and travel barriers become less of an issue. This intercultural dialogue creates a rich tapestry of herbal knowledge that cuts across national borders and advances our understanding of plant-based medicine. Traditional herbal systems, including Indigenous healing practices, TCM, and Ayurveda, offer distinctive viewpoints that contribute to the body of knowledge in herbal medicine.

A revolutionary development in the profession is the implementation of educational efforts designed to train herbalists and incorporate herbal therapy into official healthcare education programs. Educational institutions are broadening their curricula in response to the growing demand for qualified practitioners who thoroughly understand both traditional and scientific components of herbal therapy. Aspiring herbalists can acquire a foundation in plant identification, herbal preparations, and therapeutic applications through herbal medicine schools, workshops, and certifications. Herbal education is incorporated into traditional medical and healthcare training programs to promote a more patient-centered approach and give medical staff members more resources to handle various health issues.

In summary, new developments in herbal medicine show a vibrant, developing field that balances innovation and tradition. Herbal medicine is evolving to address the requirements of changing society through initiatives such as sustainable methods, individualized formulations, and botanical synergy, among other things. A more inclusive and holistic approach to well-being is fostered by the development of sustainable practices and the incorporation of herbal medicine into conventional healthcare, as scientific research on the therapeutic potential of medicinal plants continues to reveal. The combination of scientific rigor, traditional wisdom, and a dedication to tackling global health issues will shape the future of herbal therapy.

## Innovations in Botanical Research

Botanical research, a dynamic and interdisciplinary field, is experiencing a renaissance of innovation driven by technological advancements, collaborative approaches, and a deepening understanding of the intricate relationships between plants and their environments. This section delves into the most recent advances in botanical study, including molecular methods, ecological understandings, conservation tactics, and investigating plant-based applications in several domains. The field of botanical research is expanding and offers a deeper understanding of the natural world and valuable answers to global problems in environmental sustainability, agriculture, and medicine as scientists work to solve the secrets of plant life.

At the vanguard of botanical research, molecular breakthroughs are transforming our knowledge of plant biology at the genetic and biochemical levels. The quick interpretation of plant genomes and the discovery of the genetic codes governing growth, development, and responses to environmental stimuli have been made possible by developing high-throughput sequencing methods. Transcriptomics, metabolomics, and comparative genomics provide insights into the complex webs of genes and chemicals that control plant functions. Thanks to the precise genome alterations made possible by CRISPR-Cas9 gene-editing tools, there has never been more potential to engineer crops for increased resilience, nutritional value, and climatic adaptability. In addition to expanding our knowledge of fundamental biological processes, molecular advances in botanical study open the door to revolutionary new applications in biotechnological advancements, crop enhancement, and drug discovery.

Advances in ecology are transforming our understanding of plant interactions in ecosystems. At the local, regional, and global levels, remote sensing technologies—like satellite imagery and drones with sophisticated sensors—offer in-depth, non-intrusive monitoring of vegetation dynamics. Scientists may monitor changes in plant productivity, biodiversity, and reactions to environmental stressors with the help of these instruments. Effective conservation strategies are developed by examining intricate spatial patterns made more accessible by integrating remote sensing data with geographic information systems (GIS). Environmental DNA (eDNA) analysis is one of the emerging approaches transforming biodiversity assessments in terrestrial and aquatic habitats by providing non-destructive means of monitoring and identifying plant species. Integrating sophisticated modeling techniques with ecological data synthesis improves our capacity to forecast the effects of invasive species, changing land uses, and climate change on plant communities.

Revolutionary conservation biology developments use technology to protect threatened plant species and their environments. A workable method for the long-term storage of genetic material that guarantees the preservation of plant diversity and genetic resources is the cryopreservation of plant tissues, such as seeds, embryos, and meristems. Rare and endangered plant species are stored in seed banks outfitted with advanced cryopreservation methods. Furthermore, the ex-situ conservation of vulnerable plants is made possible by using tissue culture and in vitro propagation techniques, which allow for the plants' reintroduction into their natural environments. In the rapidly developing field of botanical research known as conservation genomics, genetic diversity, population dynamics, and adaption strategies of endangered plant species are evaluated using molecular methods. Combining genomics with conventional conservation methods makes conservation efforts more accurate and effective and plant populations more resilient to environmental and human stressors.

Plant-based applications are being investigated outside the traditional fields, such as pharmacy, materials science, and sustainable agriculture. Thanks to developments in analytical methods, phytochemical research reveals plants' therapeutic qualities and their possible uses in medication creation. Studies on metabolomics provide light on the wide range of secondary metabolites that plants produce and provide insights into their ecological and medicinal uses. Discovering and separating bioactive components from therapeutic plants opens the door to creating cutting-edge medications, nutraceuticals, and herbal treatments.

At the same time, advances in materials science are utilizing materials obtained from plants to create sustainable substitutes. Natural fibers, cellulose, and lignin are examples of plant-based materials being investigated for their potential uses in bioplastics, textiles, and building materials. These materials present eco-friendly substitutes for traditional synthetic goods. Using plant-derived substances in organic farming and pest control exemplifies how botanical research can support sustainable agricultural methods by lowering the need for artificial fertilizers and pesticides.

The complexities of plants' responses to environmental stimuli are revealed by plant physiology research advances, offering critical new insights into adaptations and resilience mechanisms. A rapidly developing area called "plant stress physiology" studies how plants sense and react to environmental stresses like drought, salt, and high temperatures. To design crops that can withstand pressure and implement sustainable farming practices, it is essential to comprehend the molecular and physiological mechanisms that allow some plants to flourish under challenging conditions. Plant imaging technologies, such as live-cell imaging and fluorescence microscopy, have made it possible to visualize cellular processes, growth dynamics, and interactions with symbiotic organisms in real-time. These instruments present unprecedented changes to decipher the intricacies of plant biology, ranging from the cellular and molecular processes to the synchronization of reactions throughout entire plant systems.

Transformative methods for data analysis, modeling, and prediction insights are being fostered by integrating artificial intelligence (AI) and machine learning (ML) in botanical research. Large-scale datasets are subjected to AI algorithms, which make it easier to find intricate patterns and correlations in ecological, genetic, and environmental data. Plant phenotypic classification, plant species distribution prediction, and the identification of new bioactive chemicals are all aided by machine learning algorithms. Integrating artificial intelligence (AI) with botanical research expedites the discovery rate by facilitating the extraction of significant information from extensive datasets and guiding researchers through the intricacies of plant-environment interactions. AI in plant breeding increases the effectiveness and precision of breeding programs by hastening the emergence of superior crop varieties with desired features.

Innovative studies on plant-microbe interactions can reveal the intricate links between plants and the microbial populations that live in their rhizosphere, phyllosphere, and endosphere. Analysis of microbial communities' metagenomic and metatranscriptomic regions linked to plants can shed light on their diversity and roles. Research on plant microbiomes reveals their functions in nutrition uptake, disease resistance, and stress tolerance. Using advantageous plant-microbe interactions to generate plant probiotics, biopesticides, and fertilizers that maximize crop yield while reducing environmental effects are sustainable agricultural solutions. The knowledge of how microbes affect plant health also guides the development of solutions to mitigate the impact of soil-borne diseases and increase the resilience of farming systems.

Botanical research is at the forefront of understanding and reducing the effects of changing climatic circumstances on plant communities in the context of climate change. Climate-smart agriculture refers to advancements in agricultural adaptation to changing environmental conditions. Climate-resilient farming strategies include using precision agriculture technologies, optimizing planting time, and breeding resilient crop types. Furthermore, research on climate-adaptive tactics in native plant populations contributes to the management of ecosystems and conservation initiatives. Critical knowledge is provided by research on how climate change affects plant phenology, distribution, and ecosystem dynamics to predict and mitigate the cascade impacts of climate change on biodiversity worldwide.

Technological developments in botany also encourage a more thorough investigation of the traditional plant knowledge that local and Indigenous groups possess. Ethnobotanical studies reveal the various uses of plants in medicine, traditional cultures, and sustainable resource management by bridging scientific research with traditional ecological knowledge. Respectful participation, equitable knowledge-sharing, and cultural legacy preservation are prioritized in collaborative research partnerships with Indigenous people. Traditional plant knowledge can be used in conservation plans, land-use planning, and sustainable development to help protect biodiversity and strengthen local communities.

Improvements in botanical research education are shaping the next wave of plant scientists and environmentalists. Students who enroll in interdisciplinary studies in ethnobotany, conservation biology, and plant biology will gain a comprehensive understanding of the intricacies involved in plant life. Fieldwork, cooperative research projects, and experiential learning opportunities provide students with real-world knowledge and a profound understanding of the complexities of plant ecosystems. A wider audience is involved in botanical research through digital platforms and citizen science programs, which encourage environmental stewardship and raise public understanding of the significance of plants in supporting life on Earth.

To sum up, the advancements in botanical study discussed in this section highlight how dynamic and multifaceted the area is. Botanical science is at the forefront of tackling global concerns, from ecological insights influencing conservation measures to molecular tools unlocking the genetic complexity of plant life. The breakthroughs in botanical research can potentially revolutionize sustainable agriculture, medicine, materials science, and environmental conservation as interdisciplinary collaborations grow, technology advances and our knowledge of plant-environment interactions grows. The continuous advances in botanical study provide light on the route toward a deeper understanding of the natural world and the sustainable use of its rich botanical diversity in the complex fabric of plant life.

## The Role of Botanical Defenders in Public Health

The intricate relationship between botanical defenders and public health is an evolving discourse that underscores the interconnectedness of nature and human well-being. There has been a noticeable movement in recent years to acknowledge and capitalize on the various functions plants provide to maintain public health. The multiple contributions of plant defenders are examined in this section, including ecological harmony, medical wonders, preventive power, and environmental resilience.

Ecological harmony is the basic tenet connecting botanical defenders and public health. As vital parts of ecosystems, plants significantly impact the quality of the air and water, the regulation of the climate, and biodiversity in general. Human health is greatly affected by disruptions to these botanical systems, involving anything from food security to respiratory health. A thorough grasp of the ecological interconnectedness of plants and humans demands a dedication to sustainable practices and conservation, acknowledging the innate relationship between population health and ecosystem health.

Plants have long been used for medical purposes, and this practice transcends both space and time in human society. Botanical protectors have been essential to developing therapeutic interventions for ages, from traditional herbal cures to contemporary pharmacological discoveries. This section explores the wide range of chemicals with medicinal qualities, delving into the rich pharmacopeia provided by the plant kingdom. Combining ancient knowledge with modern scientific discoveries, botanicals can treat various illnesses, from infectious diseases to chronic problems. This opens up new possibilities for drug development and innovative healthcare practices.

In addition to their medicinal uses, plant defenders significantly impact preventative healthcare. Essential nutrients and bioactive substances found in plants help to strengthen the human immune system and lower the risk of chronic illnesses. In the framework of holistic health, the section investigates the preventative potential of botanicals, examining their involvement in dietary treatments and the creation of plant-based vaccinations. Using botanicals to prevent disease aligns with a paradigm change in healthcare toward proactive approaches that put patient resilience and general well-being first when dealing with new health issues.

Resilience is demonstrated by the capacity of botanical defenders to adapt and flourish in the face of environmental difficulties. The complex methods by which plants adapt to pollution, climate change, and other stressors are examined in this section, emphasizing the significance of plant diversity preservation for environmental stability and, by extension, public health. Sustainable cohabitation requires an understanding of the interplay between ecological health and human populations since the destiny of one is inevitably connected to the fate of the other.

In summary, the story of the function of botanical defenders in public health is dynamic and ever-changing, and it merits consideration and comprehension. This section highlights the various ways that botanicals improve the health of people and communities, from the fundamentals of ecological harmony to the wonders of medicine, their ability to prevent disease, and their resilience to the environment. Taking a holistic approach that combines modern scientific discoveries with conventional knowledge is crucial for navigating the intricacies of a world that is changing quickly. In the end, appreciating and respecting the contributions made by plant defenders is essential for promoting a positive relationship between humans and the natural environment, in addition to being an issue of public health.

# CHAPTER IX

# Appendices


## Recipes for Herbal Remedies

The world of herbal remedies is a vast and rich tapestry woven from the threads of ancient traditions, cultural practices, and a deep understanding of plant properties. This section takes the reader on a tour of the world of herbalism, examining the various recipes handed down through the ages and still widely used in complementary and alternative medicine. These recipes, which range from tinctures and salves to infusions and decoctions, highlight the potential of plants to enhance health and well-being while also reflecting the diversity of healing practices across cultures.

The skill of creating infusions and decoctions is one of the fundamental tenets of herbal therapy. These preparations utilize plants' medicinal properties, whether applied topically or drunk as a comfortable tea. The section explores several techniques for making herbal infusions, such as steeping fresh or dried plant material in hot water to extract therapeutic components. Similarly, decoctioning entails simmering more fibrous plant parts, such as bark or roots, to remove their medicinal qualities. The adaptability of herbal infusions and decoctions, from chamomile tea for sleep to elderberry decoctions for immune support, is evidence of their time-tested effectiveness.

Beyond teas, concentrated herbal treatments in the form of tinctures and extracts give robust and readily quantifiable dosages. The careful method of making tinctures—in which plant material is macerated in glycerin or alcohol to extract bioactive components—is examined in this section. The need to comprehend herbal ratios and extraction techniques to get maximum effectiveness is emphasized in this section. Examples of the diversity and specificity of tinctures in addressing different health conditions range from valerian extracts for sleep support to echinacea tinctures for immunological regulation.

Herbal medicine is not limited to internal use; it also includes topical applications such as ointments and salves. This portion of the section discusses the skill of blending infused oils or essential oils with beeswax or other bases to create topical formulations. The section examines how herbalists have used plants' therapeutic qualities to treat various skin and musculoskeletal conditions, from calendula salves for skin healing to arnica ointments for muscle relaxation. How ancient knowledge and contemporary formulations work together highlights how herbal treatments are changing to fit the demands of modern patients.

Herbalism is the blending of herbs to generate synergistic combinations, where the whole is frequently more than the sum of its parts. This section delves into the idea of culinary herbalism, which turns common ingredients into powerful medicinal allies. Herbal blends for respiratory health and adaptogenic blends to boost stress resilience are just two examples of how the culinary arts include herbs to enhance the taste of herbal medicines. The section also explores how important it is to comprehend herbal tastes and energetics to customize formulations to fit each reader's unique demands and constitutions.

Indigenous knowledge and cultural traditions are closely linked with herbal treatments, representing various societies' distinct ecosystems and customs. This section discusses how different cultures have used the indigenous flora for medicinal purposes, ranging from Native American herbal traditions to Ayurvedic formulations in India. In addition to acknowledging that the recipes for herbal cures are not just about the plants themselves but also about the cultural contexts in which they flourish, it highlights the significance of honoring and protecting indigenous knowledge.

Herbal treatments provide a more comprehensive and frequently softer approach to healthcare but also present issues with standardization, regulation, and working with traditional medicine. This portion of the article looks critically at these difficulties and integration prospects in the more extensive healthcare system context. More sophisticated knowledge of the safety and effectiveness of herbal medicines is made possible by the developing field of phytotherapy and scientific studies on the subject, opening the door to compelling and knowledgeable healthcare practices.

To sum up, the realm of herbal treatments is an intriguing fabric fashioned from the strands of history, research, and cultural variety. The recipes for herbal medicines offer a sophisticated and comprehensive approach to health and well-being, ranging from the ease of use of herbal infusions to the intricacy of synergistic mixes and the profound insights of indigenous wisdom. As we traverse the potential and difficulties in herbal medicine, it is clear that the formulas passed down through the ages are dynamic and flexible, meeting the changing requirements of people and communities. By paying homage to the age-old knowledge ingrained in these formulas, we pave the way for the peaceful assimilation of herbal treatments into contemporary medicine.

## Herbal Dosage Guidelines

Navigating the world of herbal medicine requires a nuanced understanding of the diverse array of plants and the art and science of dosage. Herbal dosage recommendations carefully weigh the potential hazards against the therapeutic advantages and are the cornerstone of an effective and safe herbal treatment. The complexities of herbal dosing are examined in this section, along with the variables that affect dosage calculation, how herbal medicines are taken, and the significance of customized methods for maximizing the benefits of plant medicine.

Herbal medicine prescription is by no means a one-size-fits-all practice. This portion of the section explores the various aspects that affect the dosage of herbal remedies, from the particular qualities of the plant material to the unique traits of the patient seeking care. The potency of herbal preparations influences the intricacy of dose considerations, the variable concentrations of bioactive chemicals in various plant sections, and the intended therapeutic goals. Furthermore, the recipient's age, weight, general health, and individual sensitivities are essential for customizing herbal dosages.

There are many different types of herbal treatments, and each has other factors to consider when determining dosage. The common ways of delivering herbs, such as teas, tinctures, pills, and topical treatments, are examined in this section. Teas, derived from either fresh or dried plant matter, are a gentle and conventional method; tinctures, on the other hand, offer concentrated extracts that enable accurate dosage. For individuals who prefer a more contemporary and easily obtainable herbal medication, capsules, and tablets provide convenience and standardized dosages. Herbal dosing takes on a new level with topical treatments, including creams, salves, and poultices, which enable the targeted treatment of particular conditions.

Various medical disorders require customized methods for administering herbal remedies. This section explores how herbalists estimate proper dosages for multiple symptoms, including respiratory infections, digestive disorders, anxiety, and chronic conditions. It also examines specific criteria for common ailments. It is necessary to fully comprehend both conventional wisdom and modern scientific findings to appreciate the subtleties of herbal doses for particular illnesses. The section sheds light on how herbalists can help people find the right amounts for their specific health profiles and the subtleties of the ailments they are trying to treat.

Herbal medicine highlights the significance of customized dosage methods in light of individual differences. This section explores the need to consider an individual's lifestyle, constitution, and general health state when calculating herbal remedies dosages. The theory of constitutional herbalism emphasizes the possibility that different people may have various effects from the same herb. It is based on traditions such as Ayurveda and Traditional Chinese Medicine. Herbalists strive to maximize therapeutic results while lowering the possibility of side effects by customizing dosages of herbs to match each person's unique requirements and imbalances.

A complete awareness of the possible risks and contraindications is essential to ensuring the safety of herbal treatments. This portion of the article discusses the significance of evaluating a person's medical history, current drugs, and allergies to detect any possible interactions or negative responses. The section explores standard safety precautions, including the necessity of titrating up gradually from low doses, mainly when using solid plants. It also discusses how important it is to watch for any side effects and stop using herbs if they do.

Incorporating herbal dosages with conventional treatments is becoming increasingly crucial as herbal medicine becomes more well-recognized in the medical community. This section explores the possibilities for teamwork, highlighting the significance of communication between herbalists and traditional medical professionals. Recognizing possible conflicts between herbs and drugs, modifying dosages in response to evolving medical conditions, and encouraging candid communication among practitioners all contribute to a collaborative, holistic healthcare paradigm that maximizes the benefits of both herbal and conventional methods.

The section's concluding portion emphasizes the importance of education in enabling people to make knowledgeable judgments regarding the dosage of herbal remedies. Practitioners support a culture of ethical herbal usage by dispensing clear and accurate information. The section examines the significance of advancing self-awareness, motivating people to take an active role in their healthcare, and cultivating a feeling of accountability when it comes to herbal doses. By doing this, herbal medicine transforms into a tool for fostering a closer relationship between people and their health and a therapeutic intervention.

Finally, herbal dosage guidelines capture the delicate balance between the requirement for safety and individualization in healthcare and the powerful medicinal potential of plants. Understanding the different herbal administration methods, appreciating the complex factors that influence prescription decisions, and committing to personalized approaches that respect the individuality of each person seeking herbal support are all necessary for navigating the complex world of herbal dosing. As herbal therapy becomes increasingly integrated into contemporary healthcare, using herbal dosages responsibly becomes essential to maximizing the advantages of plant medicine while putting the health of individuals who use it first.

## Glossary of Terms

The lexicon of herbal medicine is a labyrinth of terminology that weaves traditional wisdom, botanical sciences, and holistic healthcare practices together. To create a glossary explaining the complex terminology used by herbalists and enthusiasts, this section takes readers on a tour through the rich tapestry of phrases that make up the foundation of herbalism. This thorough investigation aims to simplify herbal medicine's jargon, promoting a deeper comprehension of the fundamental ideas that guide this age-old yet rapidly developing discipline. Topics covered include botanical classifications, medicinal concepts, and preparation techniques.

Botanical nomenclature, a system of naming and classifying plants that offer a common language for communication, is the foundation of the vocabulary of herbal medicine. This section of the section explains the complexities of binomial nomenclature, in which a genus and species name are assigned to each plant. Knowing the botanical names helps with accuracy in plant identification and acts as a translator between different languages and cultures, making herbal discussions clear and accurate.

Investigating the components and phytochemistry of plants is necessary to learn more about their medicinal qualities. This section delves into the intricate realm of bioactive substances present in herbs, encompassing essential oils, glycosides, alkaloids, and flavonoids. Every component has unique qualities that contribute to a plant's medicinal actions; knowledge of phytochemistry improves one's capacity to make thoughtful herb selections based on various herbs' chemical composition and possible therapeutic benefits.

The concept of therapeutic activities and energetics, which categorizes plant effects according to their physiological consequences, is deeply ingrained in herbal therapy. This section defines terminology like nervines, adaptogens, and analgesics and provides information on how herbs can affect health. Furthermore, the section delves into the energetic properties of herbs, examining their potential to be warming or cooling, moisturizing or drying, and their impact on the body's active systems as per Ayurveda and Traditional Chinese Medicine practices.

Using different preparations and ways of administration to maximize the medicinal power of plants is part of the art of herbal medicine. This section explains the various applications of herbs for medicinal purposes, ranging from decoctions and infusions to tinctures, salves, and poultices. Knowing the subtleties of herbal preparations guarantees that practitioners and amateurs can select the best form for particular health requirements.

A key component of herbal practice is determining the

proper dosage for herbal treatments to balance safety and effectiveness. Terms associated with doses, such as tincture ratios, tea strengths, and factors to be considered for customized dosage, are discussed throughout the section. The significance of a customized approach to herbal dose is emphasized by clarifying the idea of titration, which is the process of gradually modifying dosage to determine a person's ideal therapeutic level.

A synthesis of knowledge regarding specific herbs, the Materia Medica, is fundamental to herbal education. This section delves into the botanical descriptions, historical applications, ingredients, medicinal activities, and possible contraindications of each plant profile and the terminology related to Materia Medica. Herbalists familiar with Materia Medica are better equipped to choose herbs based on each person's specific needs and health profile.

The holistic ideas that consider the connection of the

body, mind, and spirit are the foundation of herbal medicine. This section delves into concepts like vitalism, the terrain model, and holism, highlighting the significance of treating the underlying causes of imbalance instead of only treating its symptoms. The section also explores the jargon of ancient medical systems, each offering a distinct viewpoint on health and wellness, including Western herbalism, Ayurveda, and ancient Chinese Medicine.

Professional behavior and ethical issues are crucial for

people practicing therapeutic herbalism. This segment of the section delves into concepts associated with the moral application of herbal medicine, such as informed consent, maintaining client privacy, and the significance of continuous education for practitioners. The section strongly emphasizes the value of upholding honesty, openness, and respect when providing herbal consultations and the necessity of developing cooperative partnerships with other medical professionals.

Herbal medicine is praised for its mild and comprehensive approach, but recognizing some dangers and contraindications is essential. Terms like herb-drug interactions, allergic reactions, and contraindications for particular groups, including pregnant women or people with some medical issues, are explored in this section about potential dangers and safety concerns. Understanding these phrases helps one practice herbal medicine responsibly and intelligently.

Accurate plant identification is essential for the safe and efficient use of herbs. The study examines vocabulary linked to plant identification, such as phrases used in foraging, botanical keys, and plant morphology. To preserve plant populations and ecosystems, it is also essential to comprehend the fundamentals of ethical and sustainable foraging.

To sum up, this thorough examination of glossary terminology related to herbal medicine sheds light on the complex vocabulary that underpins herbal treatment. This dictionary guides navigating the complex landscape of herbalism, covering everything from the accuracy of botanical nomenclature to the subtle notions of medicinal activities, doses, and ethical considerations. Knowing this vocabulary helps people communicate more effectively. It gains a deeper grasp of the concepts that link plants' healing potential to humans as more people work with herbs and herbal medicine.

# CHAPTER X

# Resources and References

## Recommended Books and Publications

Embarking on a journey into the world of herbalism requires a connection with plants and a wealth of knowledge that spans botanical science, traditional wisdom, and clinical applications. Suggested readings and journals are essential for nourishing the herbal mind because they provide a wide range of information for novices, experts, and enthusiasts alike. The importance of carefully chosen reading lists in herbalism is examined in this section, which also highlights important works that cover the field's breadth and depth and offer insights into plant identification, therapeutic applications, medicinal qualities, and the historical and cultural backgrounds that influence herbal practices.

Herbalism is based on a profound knowledge of botany and plant identification. Suggested botanical and field guides are essential resources for anyone looking to identify and establish a connection with therapeutic plants. Readers can confidently acquire plant identification abilities with the help of thorough guides written by authors such as Michael Moore, Matthew Wood, and Thomas Elpel. These guides combine practical insights with botanical science. These publications promote a deep understanding of the plant kingdom's complexity and diversity and are helpful as reference tools.

Access to reliable and thoroughly studied references is necessary when exploring the world of medicinal plants. Textbooks written by well-known herbalists like Rosemary

Gladstar, Matthew Wood, and David Hoffmann are invaluable. These books explore the therapeutic qualities of many plants, offering comprehensive details on their components, actions as remedies, and traditional applications. These references provide a thorough basis for both herbal practitioners and amateurs, whether studying the subtleties of herbal energetics or the adaptogenic qualities of plants like Rhodiola and ashwagandha.

The foundation of herbal knowledge is Materia Medica, which provides in-depth descriptions of certain herbs. Comprehensive Materia Medica, which includes botanical descriptions, traditional usage, components, and therapeutic applications of a large variety of herbs, has been written by authors such as Michael Tierra, Matthew Wood, and David Hoffmann. These books provide a comprehensive understanding of herbal therapy by inspiring a profound appreciation for the complex relationships between people and plants and serving as selection guides for herbs.

Suggested works on clinical practice and formulation are indispensable partners for anybody pursuing clinical herbalism. With their clinical knowledge, authors such as David Winston, Thomas Easley, and Aviva Romm offer case studies, formulation techniques, and insights into herbal treatments. By bridging the gap between academic understanding and actual application, these publications enable herbalists to confidently handle complex health conditions and customize treatments to meet each patient's unique needs.

One's herbal journey gains depth when one comprehends the historical and cultural settings that influence herbal practices. Suggested readings on ethnobotany, traditional herbal remedies, and historical plant applications provide insights into how various civilizations have interacted with therapeutic plants. The accounts of writers like Stephen Harrod Buhner, Guido Mase, and Maia Toll show how herbal traditions are interwoven with human history, creating a connection between the past and present.

Specialized resources are needed to adapt herbal knowledge to particular demographics, such as older people, children, and women's health. Writers such as Susun Weed, Matthew Wood, and Aviva Romm provide advice on herbal remedies for menopause, fertility, pregnancy, and child care while also addressing the particular requirements of various demographic groups. These volumes offer a sophisticated grasp of how herbalism can be tailored to assist people's varied health journeys.

Beyond theory, herbalism includes the skills of foraging for medicinal plants and wildcrafting. James Green, Richo Cech, and Rosemary Gladstar are several authors whose books on herbal preparations are highly recommended. They walk readers through the alchemical steps of making tinctures, salves, infusions, and more. Texts on wildcrafting also shed light on sustainable harvesting methods, moral foraging techniques, and the significance of developing a mutually beneficial relationship with the land.

Herbalism and holistic health are intrinsically linked, and publications on integrative methods that are highly recommended can help build a connection between herbal remedies and other forms of therapy. Writers such as Andrew Weil, David Hoffmann, and Tieraona Low Dog offer a thorough understanding of integrative health methods and examine the connections between herbal medicine, diet, lifestyle, and traditional healthcare.

Highly suggested readings on phytochemistry, pharmacology, and evidence-based medicine become essential for anyone looking for a better scientific understanding of herbal treatment. Scholars such as Simon Mills, Kerry Bone, and Joseph Pizzorno bridge the gap between conventional wisdom and modern research by offering insights into the scientific basis of herbal therapy. These books highlight the value of evidence-based herbal therapies and add to the growing discipline of phytotherapy.

To sum up, reading suggested books and articles about herbalism opens the door to a large and constantly expanding body of information. These materials, which range from botanical guides and references to medicinal plants to clinical herbalism, cultural viewpoints, and scientific insights, all work together to feed the herbal mind and promote a comprehensive and in-depth knowledge of plant medicine. The carefully chosen reading lists provided by knowledgeable herbalists and writers serve as a light of wisdom for people just starting on their herbal journey, assisting them in navigating the maze of herbal knowledge and encouraging a lifetime dedication to the art and science of herbalism.

## Websites and Organizations for Further Exploration

The vast landscape of herbalism extends beyond the pages of books and into the digital realm, where websites and organizations serve as dynamic hubs for information, community, and ongoing exploration. In this section, we explore the various internet resources and organizational platforms that connect herbalists, lovers, and searchers of plant wisdom worldwide, thus expanding the reach of herbal knowledge. The digital world enhances the herbal journey by enabling ongoing learning, networking, and participation opportunities. These opportunities range from educational websites with in-depth articles and plant databases to groups that promote community, education, and advocacy.

For those interested in herbal remedies, a plethora of educational websites have emerged with the advent of the digital age. A wealth of articles, guides, and plant monographs can be found on websites such as Herbal Academy, The Herbalist, and Plants for a Future. These platforms, which cover subjects including herbal preparations, plant identification, and therapeutic applications, link conventional wisdom and modern findings. By using these websites, people can access a wealth of information that enables them to learn more about herbalism at their own pace.

Digital plant databases are a priceless tool for anyone looking to increase their knowledge of botany and proficiency in identification. Plant classification, distribution, and traditional usage are all covered in detail on websites such as the Missouri Botanical Garden Plant Finder, Herbal Medicine-Maker's Handbook, and the USDA Plants Database. By providing users with interactive features such as cross-referencing botanical names, exploring the diversity of the plant world, and accessing ethnobotanical material, these databases help people develop a stronger relationship with the plants that are the cornerstone of herbal therapy.

The way herbal enthusiasts interact and exchange stories has changed dramatically with the advent of digital platforms. Social media sites, forums, and online communities offer places where people may interact with other like-minded people, exchange herbal journey stories, and seek guidance. Groups on Facebook such as "Wildcrafting and Foraging" and "Herbalists Without Borders" provide a friendly environment for herbalists of all skill levels, encouraging friendship and presenting chances for collective education. These virtual platforms cut over national borders and give people access to a worldwide network of herbal wisdom and various viewpoints.

Herbal education websites provide information, webinars, and structured courses for those wishing to expand their knowledge in a more structured environment. Online courses, mentorship programs, and certification opportunities are offered by platforms such as the American Herbalists Guild, Herbal Academy, and Chestnut School of Herbal Medicine. Regardless of one's experience level, these learning environments offer flexibility and accessibility in herbal studies, making them ideal for novices and seasoned practitioners looking to further their education.

Herbalism encompasses larger-scale advocacy and research in addition to individual activities. The field is significantly advanced by groups like the American Herbalists Guild, United Plant Savers, and the National Institute of Medical Herbalists, who promote herbal medicine research and advocate for ethical wildcrafting methods and plant conservation. By being involved with these groups, people may contribute to the more extensive discussion about herbalism and its place in contemporary healthcare, in addition to having access to invaluable resources.

Digital platforms provide a voice to underrepresented voices and traditional knowledge by amplifying cultural and indigenous perspectives on herbalism. Websites such as "Ethical Wildcrafting" from United Plant Savers and "Diversity in Herbalism" from the American Herbalists Guild emphasize the significance of inclusivity and cultural competency in herbal practices. Using these resources promotes a sensitive approach to herbalism that considers the traditions of many cultures and recognizes the contributions made by indigenous people to the global body of plant knowledge.

Herbal publications and online journals provide insightful information for anyone looking for in-depth articles, research papers, and contributions from subject matter specialists. Scholarly publications, reviews, and research updates are available on platforms such as HerbalGram and the Journal of Herbs, Spices & Medicinal Plants, covering a wide range of topics from phytochemistry to clinical uses of herbal medicine. Interacting with these papers enables people to remain current on the most recent advancements in evidence-based medicine and herbal research.

With the advent of digital platforms, herbal events and conferences are now much more accessible, enabling participation from people worldwide in virtual gatherings. Attend lectures, workshops, and panel discussions with prominent herbalists at events, including the Medicines from the Earth Herb Symposium, the American Herbalists

Guild Symposium, and the International Herb Symposium. Attending these events virtually allows for continued education, networking with professionals, and exposure to various viewpoints within the herbal community.

Organizations and websites devoted to environmental conservation and sustainable practices become essential resources as more herbalists become aware of their value. The Sustainable Herbs Program, the FairWild Foundation, and United Plant Savers are devoted to supporting at-risk plant species, encouraging ethical wildcrafting, and advancing a sustainable herbal trade. By participating in these programs, herbalists can demonstrate how their activities align with ecological stewardship principles and highlight their duty to promote the preservation and well-being of the natural world.

In summary, the herbal journey becomes a dynamic and interconnected experience when websites and organizations dedicated to herbalism research are explored. The digital sphere offers ongoing education, networking, and advocacy channels, ranging from educational platforms and community spaces to plant databases and informational web pages. Interacting with these digital tools broadens personal understanding and cultivates a feeling of inclusion in the worldwide herbal community. These platforms open doors to a multitude of knowledge as we traverse the virtual terrain of herbalism, bringing us into contact with the many voices, viewpoints, and practices that contribute to the ever-changing fabric of herbal knowledge.

## References and Citations

References and citations are the pillars upon which scholarly discourse stands, grounding knowledge in a web of interconnected ideas and acknowledging the contributions of those who paved the way. In herbal literature, a thorough comprehension of references and citations indicates academic rigor and respect for the abundance of traditional wisdom, scientific discoveries, and firsthand knowledge underpinning herbalism. This section examines the significance of references and citations in herbal writing to preserve intellectual integrity, acknowledge sources, and further the continuing conversation within the herbal community.

Acknowledging sources and showing respect to the people, books, and customs that have influenced herbal knowledge is fundamental to references and citations. Herbalists can trace the genealogy of ideas and practices by referencing everything from modern scientific studies to ancient texts to classic works by renowned herbalists. It demonstrates how herbalism is linked across time and cultural boundaries and highlights the collaborative nature of knowledge creation. In addition to giving readers a path for additional exploration, citing sources promotes a culture of inquiry and respect for the various voices that weave the fabric of herbal knowledge.

Citations and references are necessary for herbal literature to retain its intellectual integrity. Authors respect integrity and openness by crediting the actual creators of ideas, concepts, and information. By ensuring that the information supplied is based on reliable sources, this dedication to intellectual honesty fosters reader trust. Academic integrity through precise and comprehensive referencing is a sign of commitment to an informed and responsible discourse in herbal literature, where combining traditional wisdom and scientific understanding is vital.

Herbalism is a dynamic field that thrives on ongoing discussion, combining established wisdom and newfound understanding. Citations and references give readers entrance points into this discussion and enable them to examine how concepts and methods have changed. Herbal literature embodies herbalism's dynamic and adaptable nature by referencing historical writings and modern studies. In addition to adding to their personal story, authors contribute to the larger discourse in the herbal community, which encourages a cooperative idea- sharing environment and broadens the group's comprehension of plant medicine.

A broad spectrum of genres and readers are covered by herbal literature, ranging from traditional writings with folklore roots to scholarly articles published in peer-reviewed publications. The range of citation styles used reflects the diversity of herbal literature. Traditional herbalists may consult oral traditions, ethnobotanical techniques, and lineage-based teachings, but academic journals may follow rigorous citation styles like APA, MLA, or Chicago style. It takes flexibility and a sophisticated awareness of the target audience to navigate several citation styles and ensure that the selected format adheres to academic norms and genre conventions.

The honorable and moral citation of traditional and indigenous knowledge is a distinctive feature of herbal literature. Herbal techniques are based on the wisdom of indigenous cultures and traditional healers, whose contributions must be acknowledged. When citing sources of conventional knowledge, authors should exercise cultural awareness, obtain permission when needed, and refrain from exploitation or appropriation. Citing traditional and indigenous knowledge needs to be more than just a formality; it should represent a dedication to acknowledgment, reciprocity, and the conservation of cultural legacy.

Herbal literature frequently combines scientific information from recent research and anecdotal evidence gleaned from centuries of traditional use. To reference effectively, writers must assiduously combine the two forms of evidence, appreciating the importance of past customs while embracing the developments of contemporary science. In addition to enhancing the breadth of herbal literature, balancing anecdotal and scientific references helps close the gap between conventional and evidence-based methods, promoting an integrative and holistic viewpoint.

Certain aspects of herbalism, especially those involving lesser-known plants or traditional medicines, provide a particular reference issue due to the scarcity of study. Although there may not always be a substantial body of data supporting every herbal remedy in scientific literature, authors can overcome this difficulty by openly recognizing the limits and combining traditional knowledge, clinical experience, and accessible research. This method fosters a modest acknowledgment of the knowledge gaps in the field while promoting further investigation and study in less-traveled herbalism domains.

The foundation of ethical herbal literature is the appropriate citation and reference of sources, emphasizing integrity, authenticity, and a dedication to the welfare of readers and the larger herbal community. By properly crediting their sources, offering easily accessible references for readers to investigate further, and treating traditional knowledge with cultural sensitivity, authors contribute significantly to advancing ethical behavior. The honest literature on herbal medicine is distinguished by its commitment to openness, recognition of many perspectives, and deliberate attempts to contribute to the current conversation within the herbal community.

Finally, citations and references serve as the framework for herbal writing, tying together the various experience, science, and tradition strands. They must play the tasks of recognizing sources, upholding intellectual integrity, fostering ethical behavior, and contributing to continuing discourse. The need for authors to understand different citation styles, honor traditional and indigenous knowledge, and handle research obstacles grows as herbalism develops and appeals to a worldwide readership. Herbal literature becomes a dynamic and inclusive environment that respects the origins of herbal wisdom while promoting a cooperative and constantly expanding dialogue within the herbal community by preserving the standards of scholarly practice and ethical conduct.

# CONCLUSION

### Recap of Key Takeaways

Embarking on the journey of herbal exploration reveals a vast and intricate landscape of knowledge, where the roots of tradition intertwine with the branches of contemporary understanding. A few essential lessons become apparent as we explore the herbal world, influencing how we view the comprehensive and complex field of plant medicine. The fundamental aspect of herbalism is, first and foremost, the understanding of plants as dynamic living entities with individual spirits and energies. This viewpoint encourages us to treat herbal treatments with respect and a profound awareness of the connections between plant life and people.

Herbalism's cornerstones are the significance of plant identification and moral foraging practices. Acquiring the ability to identify, respect, and responsibly gather medicinal plants is essential for their preservation and is the foundation for making powerful and efficient herbal treatments. Herbalists become stewards of biodiversity by developing a bond with the earth and the plants there, incorporating moral behavior into their work.

Herbal energetics is rooted in traditional medical systems like Ayurveda and Traditional Chinese Medicine. It adds a new perspective on the properties of plants and how they affect human health. Herbalists can customize treatments to individual constitutions by understanding the warming or cooling nature, moistening or drying properties, and general energetics of herbs. This allows them to create a harmonious balance that aligns with each person's needs.

Herbalists have a wide range of options when creating treatments that address particular health issues and personal preferences thanks to the art of herbal preparations, which includes infusions, decoctions, tinctures, and salves. Herbal therapies are characterized by their versatility and applicability to various health concerns. Each preparation process offers a unique way to extract and preserve the therapeutic components of plants.

Comprehending the recommended dosage for herbs becomes essential to responsible and productive use. A balance between therapeutic advantages and safety is ensured by considering aspects such as the potency of herbal preparations, age, weight, and general health of the individual when determining dosage. The idea of titration emphasizes the value of individualized approaches in herbal therapy by progressively changing dosage to determine each person's ideal therapeutic level.

Herbalism incorporates various indigenous knowledge and cultural customs beyond individual practices. To navigate the herbal environment responsibly, respect for different perspectives and acceptance of traditional knowledge are essential. It takes cultural competence, sensitivity, and awareness of possible appropriation to create a harmonious blend of ancient and modern herbal methods.

A cooperative approach is necessary to integrate herbal therapy into contemporary healthcare systems. A more comprehensive knowledge of the safety and effectiveness of herbal remedies is made possible by the developing field of phytotherapy, supported by scientific studies on the subject. Open communication, awareness of potential herb-drug interactions, and encouraging cooperative partnerships between herbal practitioners and conventional healthcare providers are critical in bridging the gap between herbal and traditional treatment.

Authors who successfully negotiate the challenges of referencing and citations demonstrate the importance of responsible herbal writing in printed and digital formats. Essential components of ethical herbal literature include acknowledging sources, upholding intellectual integrity, and participating in the continuing discussion within the herbal community. Herbal literature gains authenticity and credibility when different citation formats are used, study limitations are addressed, and respectful reference to traditional and indigenous knowledge is encouraged.

Herbal knowledge is a living tapestry from scientific, traditional, and cultural variations. Herbal medicine's major lessons encourage us to approach plants humbly and acknowledge their innate wisdom and capacity for healing. We become more than just practitioners when we embrace moral behavior, promote cultural sensitivity, and navigate the intricate network of herbal knowledge; we become custodians of a legacy that reaches well beyond our own. These essential lessons are a foundation for our continued exploration of herbalism, helping mold our path toward a more sustainable and all-encompassing approach to health and well-being.

## Empowering Readers to Embrace Herbal Antivirals

In the face of global health challenges, the exploration and embrace of herbal antivirals emerge as a compelling avenue for individuals seeking to enhance their well- being. With its roots in ancient customs and growing scientific knowledge, the field of herbalism provides a wide range of plant companions with antiviral qualities. By examining the fundamentals of herbal antivirals, investigating the processes by which plants display antiviral activity, highlighting essential herbs in this category, and offering helpful advice on incorporating herbal antivirals into regular wellness routines, this section seeks to empower readers.

A subclass of plant medicine called herbal antivirals is dedicated to treating viral infections. Understanding the fundamental ideas driving their action is essential to appreciating their efficacy. Herbs that are antiviral function in multiple ways, including preventing the growth of viruses, adjusting the immune system, and having direct virucidal properties. The antiviral activities of these herbs are attributed to the presence of bioactive components, including flavonoids, polyphenols, alkaloids, and essential oils. Furthermore, several herbs have immune-modulating properties that strengthen the body's defenses against viral invaders. Combining these processes highlights the diverse range of actions that herbal antivirals can take to help the body fight and resist viral infections.

Many different types of herbs have gained popularity due to their antiviral solid qualities. One well-known example is echinacea, prized for its immune-stimulating properties, especially against respiratory viruses. The flavonoids quercetin and anthocyanins found in elderberries have antiviral properties, especially against influenza viruses. With solid roots in Traditional Chinese Medicine, astragalus has immune-modulating properties that help the body fight off viral infections. Strong virucidal qualities make antiviral essential oils—like eucalyptus and tea tree oil—valuable for topical treatments and aromatherapy. These herbs add only a tiny portion of the enormous pool of plant allies with antiviral potential, each bringing particular advantages to the herbalist's toolkit.

Giving readers practical advice on incorporating these plants into regular wellness routines is essential to inspiring them to embrace herbal antivirals. Antiviral herbs can be added to one's routine using herbal teas, tinctures, and decoctions. For example, making tea with elderberry, echinacea, and astragalus offers a tasty and energizing drink. Concentrated liquid extracts called tinctures provide a robust and easy-to-administer herbal medication option with an accurate dose. Furthermore, adding antiviral herbs to food preparations—garlic, thyme, or oregano, for example—improves flavor and strengthens the immune system. Topical treatments, including herbal salves or essential oil blends, provide focused assistance for viral skin issues.

Herbal antivirals are frequently most effective when used with other formulations that work well together. To develop comprehensive formulations, herbalists often blend immune-modulating and adaptogenic allies with antiviral plants. For example, a well-rounded approach to viral resilience can be achieved by combining immune-supportive herbs like holy basil and adaptogens like ashwagandha with antiviral herbs like lemon balm, thyme, and licorice root. Synergistic formulations acknowledge the interdependence of the immune system, stress response, and general well-being, considering the holistic aspect of health.

Encouraging readers to use herbal antivirals goes beyond prescribing specific treatments and instead emphasizes building comprehensive immune support. The main pillars of immunological resilience are stress management, nutrition, and lifestyle choices. A key component of holistic wellness is promoting a diet high in nutrients and full of foods that strengthen the immune system, such as fruits, vegetables, and herbs. Immune support includes getting enough sleep, staying hydrated, and exercising regularly. Because of the significant adverse effects of stress on immunological function, herbalists frequently stress the value of reducing stress through exercises like yoga, meditation, and mindfulness. People can cultivate a robust and resilient immune system by integrating herbal medicines with holistic lifestyle choices.

Herbal antivirals are a great way to promote immune function, but using them should be done so mindfully and with awareness. Comprehending personal medical histories, possible contraindications, and the significance of dosage calculations constitute conscientious herbal medicine's fundamental component. Some plants could interfere with prescription drugs, and others might not be appropriate for people with certain medical conditions.

When introducing potent antiviral herbs into their regimens, pregnant women and those with long-term medical conditions should proceed cautiously and consult trained herbalists or specialists. A comprehensive and well-informed wellness strategy also benefits from acknowledging the significance of diversity in one's approach to health, which includes speaking with medical professionals and keeping lines of communication open.

Encouraging readers to use herbal antivirals requires a dedication to continuous learning and cooperation. Whether through books, online classes, or seminars, herbal education equips people with the information and abilities needed to choose wisely when it comes to herbal therapies. Working together with licensed herbalists, medical professionals, and other wellness practitioners enhances the effectiveness of a multidisciplinary approach by bringing together the advantages of several modalities. Understanding the dynamic nature of herbalism and how it fits into traditional healthcare calls for an open mind, a curious attitude, and a readiness to embark on a lifetime learning process.

In summary, enabling readers to use herbal antivirals represents a voyage into the core of plant medicine, where history and research come together to promote immunological resilience. The foundation for an all-encompassing approach to well-being is laid by comprehending the fundamentals of herbal antivirals, investigating essential herbs, including these plants in routine wellness routines, and appreciating the significance of holistic immune support. Cautionary and thoughtful remarks highlight the necessity of responsible herbal practice, stressing customized strategies and cooperative interaction with medical specialists. The importance of herbal education and cooperation becomes clear as readers navigate this terrain, encouraging a constant flow of information and a shared dedication to holistic health. Those who embrace the wisdom of herbal antivirals walk a path that promotes their health and helps them connect to the rich tapestry of plant medicine, where traditional knowledge and modern understanding converge in a harmonious dance of resilience and healing.

## Looking Ahead: Your Journey with Botanical Defenders

Embarking on a journey with botanical defenders heralds a captivating exploration into the vast and dynamic world of plant medicine. The botanical defenders welcome you to this world of whispering old traditions and resonant modern ideas. They are allies and mentors, lending their knowledge to anybody looking to improve their well-being by utilizing the transforming power of plants. This section is like a beacon, showing us the way forward, full of opportunities, revelations, and a deep connection to the floral tapestry that envelops us.

The understanding that plants are living, thinking, dynamic entities is the foundation of your adventure with botanical guardians. In contrast to inert substances, these botanical partners carry life forces and energy essences that interact with the human body on physical, emotional, and spiritual levels. The first step in the trip is to develop a profound sense of reverence and respect for the plant kingdom, realizing that humans and plants have a symbiotic relationship that has developed over thousands of years. Approach these defenders as co-creators in the complex dance of healing rather than just as people who need to be healed when you interact with them.

Plant identification develops into a fundamental ability that personally invites you to know the botanical world. Gaining the capacity to differentiate between different plants and identify minute differences in their development patterns, leaves, and flowers can provide you with much botanical knowledge. Along the way, field guides, plant identification apps, and the guidance of knowledgeable herbalists prove to be important allies. You will learn about the distinctive qualities of each plant as well as their traditional applications, folklore, and the cultural fabric they weave through this process.

Sustainable gathering methods and ethical foraging become guiding concepts that promote a mutually beneficial relationship with the land and its flora. Whether in cultivated gardens or untamed areas, the botanical defenders join together to promote conservation and cohabitation. Comprehending the seasonal patterns of plants, honoring their life cycles, and leaving offerings of appreciation behind are all components of mindful harvesting. Adopting ethical foraging practices helps preserve plant diversity and the fragile ecosystems supporting flora and fauna.

The study of herbal energetics offers a more complex perspective on the properties of plants and how they affect human health. Every botanical defense has a distinct energy signature that can either moisturize or dry, warming or chilling. Herbal energetics explores the relationship between plants and the body's constitution, enabling you to customize treatments to meet specific needs. This personalized method, which has its roots in age-old practices like Traditional Chinese Medicine and Ayurveda, encourages you to align your herbal practice with the dynamic interaction of energies inside and outside yourself.

As a creative manifestation of your journey with plant defenders, the art of herbal concoctions emerges. The endless possibilities range from making nourishing herbal tinctures and teas to creating calming salve mixes and fragrant essential oil mixtures. Making herbal medicine changes how you interact with your botanical allies by transforming commonplace components into powerful cures that capture the wisdom and intention in their preparation. Engaging in hands-on activities at the pharmacy can help you connect with the healing potential of plants on a practical level.

A crucial component of ethical herbal therapy is dosage considerations, which help you balance safety and efficacy. Comprehending the potency and suitable dosage of herbal remedies conforms to the concepts of comprehensive well-being. Herbalists frequently discuss titration, which is the process of gradually adjusting dosage to determine each person's ideal therapeutic level. This subtle method fosters a smooth integration of botanical defenders into your well-being journey by emphasizing monitoring the body's responses and modifying remedies accordingly.

The complex tapestry woven by cultural and historical viewpoints strengthens your relationship with botanical defenders. You engage in conversation with the wisdom of ancestors' knowledge as you dig into plant customs and folklore. The fact that you are aware of the cultural significance and historical use of plants adds to the experience's complexity. These viewpoints, which cover Native American herbalism, European herbal traditions, or indigenous civilizations' medical practices, provide insights that cut across time and deepen your knowledge of the plant allies.

Your experience with botanical defenders goes beyond individual health, including community and the world's connectivity. Herbalism as a communal practice encourages cooperation, knowledge sharing, and celebrating different viewpoints. Through collective wisdom, community herbalism becomes a force for good, empowering both individuals and communities. Your journey becomes essential to a more enormous, transformational tapestry as you engage in conversations about botanical defenders, share your experiences, and learn from others.

Incorporating botanical defenses into contemporary healthcare systems highlights how herbalism's role in tackling today's health issues is evolving. Understanding the possible synergies between conventional medicine becomes crucial as you negotiate this confluence. A holistic paradigm of wellness incorporates open communication, teamwork with healthcare practitioners, and an informed approach. Your journey links the cutting-edge advances in contemporary healthcare and the age-old wisdom of botanical defenders, encouraging a more inclusive and holistic approach to wellness.

Continuous education is a compass, directing your route with the most recent understandings, findings, and research in herbal medicine. Whether via books, seminars, workshops, or mentoring, the quest for knowledge develops into a lifetime endeavor. Since the world of botany is constantly changing, keeping up with the latest developments enables you to modify and improve your work while expanding your knowledge of botanical defenders and their numerous benefits to well-being.

Imagine a landscape beyond time and space as you plan your next steps with the botanical defenders. Your investigation into plant medicine establishes a connection between you and the knowledge of previous generations, the rich fabric of the present, and the possibility of future healing and transformation. Walk the route with botanical allies by your side, and embrace the delights and trials, the discoveries and secrets. Your journey with botanical defenders is a celebration of the interdependent web of life, wherein the ever-expanding tendrils of your personal experiences, the branches of modern knowledge, and the roots of tradition merge in a healing, resilient, and empowering dance.

*Thank you for buying and reading/listening to our book. If you found this book useful/helpful please take a few minutes and leave a review on the platform where you purchased our book. Your feedback matters greatly to us.*

Printed in the USA
CPSIA information can be obtained
at www.ICGtesting.com
CBHW071237140724
11413CB00023B/924